# FATTY LIVER

## DIET COOKBOOK

*A Liver Cleanse And Detox Guide: Lose Weight Fast, Improve Health And Live Longer By Burning Stubborn Fat. Complete Shopping List For The 21 Days Meal Prep Included!*

## PAULINE ANDERSON

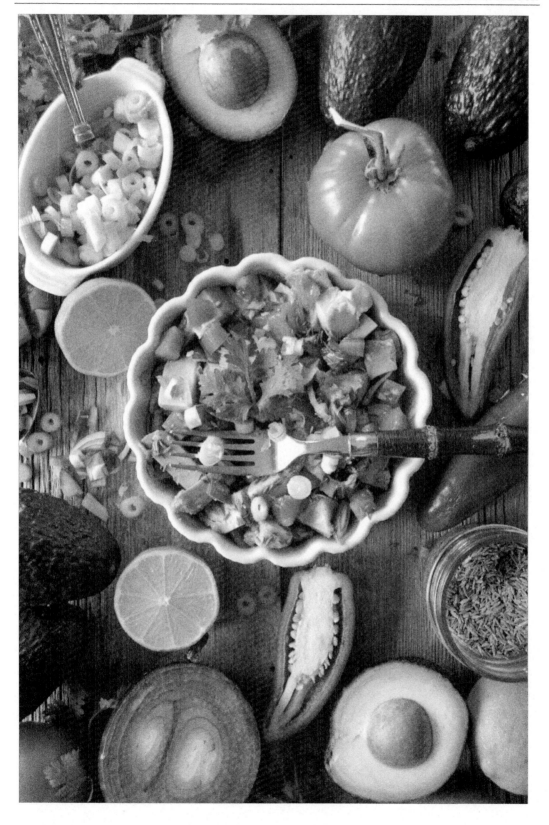

## DISCLAIMER
### THIS BOOK DOES NOT PROVIDE ANY MEDICAL ADVICE

The information contained on this book is for informational purposes only. No material on this book is intended to be a substitute for professional medical advice, diagnosis or treatment. Always seek the advice of your physician or other qualified health care provider with any questions you may have regarding treatment and before undertaking a new health care regimen.

# Table Of Contents

**CHAPTER 11: SHAKE AND SMOOTHIE RECIPES................................................76**

# CHAPTER 1: My Success Story

I'm not a health guru, a salesperson, or a healer. I'm a normal person, who like you has a fervent desire for a happy and healthy life. Here's my story.

First and foremost I'm a wife and the mother of a wonderful family and my profession is dietician.

I've always been a balanced person with a sunny disposition, loving life, food, and cooking, with a healthy marriage as well, and proud to have two wonderful children.

I've always loved to cook, pouring my enthusiasm into my family's enjoyment and tending to their needs.

But I haven't always had an easy life, suffering from various health and digestive problems and anxiety, with bad eating habits and deleterious food choices.

Practically without realizing it, stress and the lack of physical activity led me to nutritional imbalance and incessant weight gain, until I finally found myself weighing over 190 lbs.

Suffering from continual stomach problems, high blood pressure, and blood sugars, I found myself sick and worried about my health and generally dissatisfied with my life. I felt ungainly, overweight and unsightly, but could not stop eating certain foods. I felt inadequate in my energies toward my children and generally suffered feelings of frustration and anger.

Needless to say, my favorite clothes were no longer fit and physical activity was more than exhausting! Along with this loss of self-esteem, I was aware that my husband seemed to be losing interest in me.

On May 4, 2017, after liver pains, I was diagnosed as having NAFLD, with inflammation and fibrosis and risking steatohepatitis. I was angry, but very frightened a well.

Ultimately, this anger and the love of life and the love for my family fueled me and gave me impetus to find the strength to react .... All this had to change! I was determined to take control of my life and the responsibility regarding my health!

From that moment on and for the last 3 years, I have placed every effort and all my willpower and unshakable commitment in finding the path back to good health.

I have studied the matter in-depth, consulted other specialists, determined the most appropriate exercise workouts, dietary and nutritional models for weight loss and for reestablishing liver health. (These last are inextricably connected). I have gained experience and assimilated information in these last few years as never before.

But above all, I have tested and found the combinations for the healthiest cooking solutions.

I have explored alternatives to modern medicine, tried nutritional supplements and products, and explored the best methods for liver detoxification.

So in my mind, "the trick is finding the right combination and balance between the right food, physical exercise, and the best routine and method for liver detox ". And I think I've found it!

As of the present, I no longer have a fatty liver. My digestive problems have disappeared and all my blood levels are normal once again. I've lost 60 lbs. and I feel better than before, happy again

I'm staying in shape with regular physical activity and have learned to eat well, but above all, to live well.

I feel like a super mom, in great shape and I'm once more wearing my favorite outfits, desirable in my husband's eyes the way things used to be.

And I want you to be able to experience the same success!

And finally, I decided to share this with you.

With this volume you will have purchased an access to my personal experience and all the information that has given me such encouraging results, including many delicious and simple recipes and secrets that I have discovered along the way.

You will be able to maintain a healthy liver the way I have and be pleased with what you see in the mirror while at the same time discovering the joy of healthy nutrition for your liver. But remember, you will need a commitment that comes from the determination to follow the book's indications.

## PAULINE'S RECOMMENDATIONS:

Given that none of us are the same, choose the suggestions best suited for you in reading this book. Be open to advice and alternatives, always monitoring your health, exams, and confronting your experience and results with your M.D. But remember to maintain a balanced, critical mind about inauspicious diagnoses, ones that tend to be hopeless or that resemble a sentence of doom. Our bodies are marvelous machines with a wonderful capacity for self-healing. And when we do the right thing, we can activate this power.

Have moderation with the right food and limit sugars, and in this book you will find a quantity of nutritional choices. Stay active, be happy and optimistic, and with your efforts, the results will be inevitable.

Be curious and take the time you need because big results are made with small daily gestures repeated over time. And if you will let me, through this book I'll accompany you along the way.

"Pauline, after the love and passion placed in developing this book, promises those who have shown their trust by purchasing it, to update it periodically with new tips, information, activities, and recipes, and is happy to accept suggestions and feedback from all those who have placed their trust in it. More than just buying a book, this is acquiring a course that is being continually updated."

For chat, or any suggestions, feedback, review or help, please don't hesitate to contact me at my email: p.anderson.customerscare@gmail.com

If you like the book, please don't hesitate to leave a review on Amazon. Thank you and have a happy life.

# CHAPTER 2:

# What Exactly is a Fatty Liver?

Y ou are probably thinking: "Fatty liver? What does that even mean?" Fatty liver literally means that you have excess fat in your liver. You may have also heard it referred to as hepatic steatosis. Put simply, it occurs when the liver cells, known as hepatocytes, become so filled with fat that it affects their ability, and therefore the liver's ability, to function effectively.

Your liver is like a factory that never sleeps. As we discussed in earlier chapters, the liver is divided into three functioning parts: the processing plant, the distribution center, and the storehouse. As your liver processes the blood that it receives from the body, it breaks down the nutrients from your food and distributes these vital nutrients back to the rest of your body so it can better absorb them. These nutrients help to make the blood plasma proteins and other key elements that are helpful in aiding digestion. The liver will hold on to any extra nutrients that you do not need to use right away and store them safely for future use. It also processes any toxins entering your body through your food and is able to eliminate them before they can harm you.

When your liver is functioning efficiently, it is the major fat burning organ in your body and is able to pump excessive fat within your body out through the bile and excrete it as feces. While a healthy liver will help keep your weight under control, an unhealthy liver will cause fat to build up in your liver and in the rest of your body. Your liver itself will become swollen and full of toxic fat.

This begins to block the pathways that blood normally flows along and makes it difficult for the blood to be cleansed properly. When this happens, the blood that is returning to the heart is full of unhealthy fats and toxins and can damage your heart, and immune system as well.

When your liver becomes overwhelmed with too many toxins and fatty cells over time, it ceases to be able to do its job.

It cannot function properly and this causes a backup in the liver. It also means that your blood will not circulate properly, important nutrients cannot be delivered to other vital organs, and your body cannot detoxify naturally, so even more toxins will build up in your liver.

This vicious cycle is the result of fatty liver disease and it needs to be addressed by crucial lifestyle changes to prevent even more serious, and potentially fatal, health complications from arising.

## Functions of The Liver

In general, liver has approximately 500 different functions. Some of the important functions of liver are listed below:

- Responsible for processing the food once it has been digested.
- Cleans and filters the blood.
- Produces bile that aids the digestion of lipids in the small intestine.
- Maintains and produces the hormone balance in our body.
- Produces proteins and enzymes that aid in chemical reactions in the body, for example, blood clotting and repairing tissue.
- Safeguards us by fighting infections and diseases.
- Responsible for destroying and deal with harmful chemicals such as drugs or poisons.
- Helps in controlling the amount of cholesterol.
- Stores and releases tremendous amount of energy that can be used rapidly when the body needs it most.
- Stores minerals vitamins, sugars and iron.
- The greatest of all is that our liver repairs damage and renews itself.

## Latest Research

There has been a bunch of studies throughout the emergence of liver diseases to understand more about how these diseases start, how they function and how to potentially correct them. One such study was published in Auton 2019 called Effects of Periodic Fasting and Fatty Liver. It was conducted as a prospective observational study of 697 patients. The study used a mixture of patients limited by a suspected fatty liver condition and others who had a definitive fatty liver. 364 patients had a fatty liver with an index higher than 60, 38 of which were also diabetic type 2. They used this large collective as they wanted to measure and regulate the fatty liver index progression and what the index was before evolving into liver cirrhosis.

The study showed that there are not many treatments for fatty liver, and it is asymptomatic at the beginning, so the people don't notice they have the problem. It comes from overeating, consuming an excess of carbohydrates and especially fructose, while not doing enough exercise. Once establishing this, they set out to see what the impact of adding in the elements of a fast would be on the condition.

When you fast, you lose fat not only in your abdomen but all over the body. It also aids in sending down the triglycerides in your bloods. Due to this metabolism uses fat as fuel so it's very normal that the body tries to find the fat available throughout the body. It first looks in the blood, both in the tissues and of course in the liver.

So how can we understand what this index is made of, to control it? The fatty liver index is made up of four parameters. The first one is a liver enzyme called the gamma D T. Gamma DT is an enzyme that comes up when the liver suffers or is inflamed. The amount of Gamma DT reduces during a fast.

The second parameter of this index is the circumference of the abdomen. When we lose fat in the abdomen, the likelihood of this progressing decreases. The third index occurs based on the blood lipid and the rate at which the triglycerides go down. The last parameter is based on your BMI which is a reflection of your entire body weight so that all index is going down.

Understanding how the fatty liver index could be an extraordinary opportunity for people suffering from fatty liver that they don't evolute in these more severe stages which are sometimes not reversible anymore.

## Relationship Between Fatty Liver Diet And Keto Diet

Ketogenic diet is an effective treatment for nonalcoholic fatty liver disease (NAFLD). Nonalcoholic fatty liver disease (NAFLD) is a major cause of chronic liver disease, characterized by hepatic fat accumulation and possible development of inflammation, fibrosis, and cancer. The ketogenic diet (KD), with its drastic carbohydrate reduction, is a now popular weight loss intervention, despite safety concerns on a possible association with fatty liver. However, KDs were also reported to be beneficial on hepatic pathology, with ketone bodies recently proposed as effective modulators of inflammation and fibrosis. If the beneficial impact of weight loss on NAFLD is established, less is known on the effect of macronutrient distribution on such outcome. In a hypocaloric regimen, the latter seems not to be crucial, whereas at higher calorie intake, macronutrient ratio and, theoretically, ketosis, may become important. KDs could positively impact NAFLD for their very low carbohydrate content, and whether ketosis plays an additional role is unknown. Indeed, several mechanisms may directly link ketosis and NAFLD improvement, and elucidating these aspects would pave the way for new therapeutic strategies. We herein aimed at providing an accurate revision of current literature on KDs and NAFLD, focusing on clinical evidence, metabolic pathways involved, and strict categorization of dietary interventions.

# CHAPTER 3:

# What are the 4 Stages of Cirrhosis of the Liver?

**Liver Cirrhosis occurs in stages. Namely:**

Stage One: Inflammation:

The first sign of liver disease is inflammation which causes it to be slightly enlarged and tender. Inflammation is usually a sign that your body is employing its natural defense tactics to fight an infection, heal injury or any foreign intrusion to restore health.

However, if inflammation keeps getting triggered by what is attacking your liver the damage becomes more than the benefit and can result in serious damage to your liver. The tricky thing about liver inflammation is that unlike most other inflammations that will give you a sign that there is inflammation through redness, pain or elevated temperature; it does not give any form of discomfort and therefore it becomes very difficult to identify liver inflammation.

If, however, your doctor is able to identify inflammation in your liver during a routine checkup, it becomes very easy to stop the problem that could be causing this in its tracks before it progresses and causes serious damage to your liver. It is therefore important to schedule routine checkups.

**Stage Two: Scarring or Fibrosis**

When inflammation is not identified, it leads to scarring that's literally formed every time the inflammation goes down only to come back again and again, considering how tender the liver is. This scarring when uncontrolled continues growing to the point that it now replaces what used to be your healthy liver tissue. The bad thing about this is the fact that scarred tissue cannot do the same work that your previously healthy liver tissue could. As more and more of fibrosis occurs, your liver tissue starts losing sensitivity and its functions start getting impaired as it has to work many times harder than it should to get a simple function done.

If you are able to get an accurate diagnosis at this stage, your doctor will prescribe medication and a lifestyle change that will restore your liver to health in a relatively short duration.

**Stage Three: Cirrhosis**

Cirrhosis is the complete scarring of your entire liver, replacing the soft liver tissue with hard scar tissue. The liver will struggle and push to carry out its functions but if not treated will fail and not be able to work effectively or in the worst-case scenario, will not be able to work at all.

This is where the symptoms start being visible. Once you start experiencing the symptoms we outlined earlier, it is important that you seek medical help immediately! Once you get the proper diagnosis, your doctor will fast focus on containing the disease, so it does not progress. Once this has been achieved, the focus will shift to restoration which will be a deliberately slow process to ensure the damage is not exacerbated.

**Stage Four: ESLD (End Stage Liver Disease)**

At this stage, your liver is fully done in and there is very little chance of reversal as decompensation has occurred and the only option is a liver transplant. Decompensation usually includes an impairment of your kidney function, encephalopathy, lung problems, variceal bleeding and fluid retention in your abdomen that has to be physically drained. For this reason, such a patient is given priority in the liver transplant list.

# What Prescription Drugs Can Cause Cirrhosis?

Some prescription drugs can induce a version of cirrhosis known as Alcohol Cirrhosis or other chronic liver disease. Some of these medications include:

- Rheumatrex (methotrexate)
- Cordarone (amiodarone)
- Aldomet (methyldopa)

## How to Manage Symptoms

The symptoms are going to vary depending on what stage of cirrhosis you are in. At onset, there may be very little or no symptoms at all but then with the disease progression, you could start experiencing:

- Abnormally itchy skin
- Extreme sudden weight gain or weight loss
- Edema (fluid retention) manifesting as swollen legs, ankles and abdomen
- Traces of blood in your stool
- Extreme fatigue
- Dark brown or orange colored urine
- Loss of appetite
- Jaundice that manifests as the yellowing of the whites of your eyes or skin
- Light-colored stool (pointing to insufficient bilirubin)
- Unexplained bruising
- Sudden personality changes that include disorientation and confusion

One of the earliest signs of cirrhosis is edema which is basically retention of salt and fluid. It often manifests as a slightly swollen leg or ankle at first. With time, the fluid retention extends to your abdomen, a condition known as ascites. When identified early, your doctor will advise you to reduce your intake of salt and also prescribe diuretics. However, if you have a severe case of ascites, your doctor may need to drain the fluid. This is because if the fluid is not drained it could lead to an infected abdomen, referred to as peritonitis.

If left unattended to and the fluid retention continues to the point it does not respond to any form of treatment, it could lead to the need of a liver transplant.

So, how do you manage or treat liver cirrhosis?

Although there is no full cure of cirrhosis of the liver, there are treatments and management procedures that help in delaying its progress and reducing its symptoms and in so doing reduce the complications that come with liver disease and reduce the damage done to the liver cells.

- Fluid retention in joints and the abdomen is first managed by following a very low sodium diet. For extreme cases of ascites, the doctor may have to drain the fluid from your stomach. Diuretics may also be prescribed to help reduce the fluid buildup.

- If a patient's cirrhosis is as a result of excessive alcohol consumption, then the first step is to refrain from any alcohol intake. This gives the liver a chance to take a break from the detoxification of toxins brought about by alcohol.

- A healthy, low sodium and balanced diet with recommended drug therapy can be used to help improve the disorientation and confused mental conditions of patients. In some cases, laxatives may be prescribed to help absorb toxins thus reducing the liver's job.

- A lifestyle change that includes a healthy and natural low sodium diet and regular physical activity is recommended to all patients as it help the body heal itself by tapping into its primal self-healing ability.

- For cirrhosis that was exacerbated by underlying medical conditions such as autoimmune diseases, the doctor will start by addressing the underlying conditions and in cases where the damage was not too much, the damage can actually be reversed.

- Patients with severe cirrhosis may need to get a liver transplant when all forms of treatment do not respond, and the damage of the liver continues worsening.

- In cases of autoimmune hepatitis, the patient will be prescribed for drugs that suppress the immune system such as azathioprine.

- For hemochromatosis patients, treatment will involve removing blood in order lower iron levels thus preventing further liver damage. In cases of Wilson's disease where there is excess copper in the blood and liver, drugs will be administered to increase the removal of copper from the body through the urine.

- Do not use non-steroidal anti-inflammatory medication. These include naproxen and ibuprofen. This is because patients with cirrhosis of the liver can further damage their livers and kidneys with such drugs.

- Individualized treatment of patients with hepatitis C. the reason for this is that not all patients are in a position to receive antiviral treatment as it could lead to further liver damage for some people. A doctor specializing in liver disease will carry out a series of tests to determine the best course of treatment.

- Vaccinating patients with cirrhosis against hepatitis A and B infections. This helps prevent further damage to the liver.

## Using Diet to Manage Cirrhosis and Chronic Liver Diseases

Cirrhosis is a condition which makes your liver stop working properly and also affects its ability to release glycogen, a chemical which is required to provide energy to your body when you need it. When liver is not able to release glycogen, your body starts using its own muscle tissues to provide energy. A situation like this can lead to conditions like malnutrition, weakness and muscle wasting.

If your condition worsens and progresses to cirrhosis, you need to be very careful with your diet. You would need a diet that supports your liver function and also can save you from malnutrition. The best way is to immediately approach a certified doctor or dietician for a strategically designed diet plan.

Let's now talk about various types of cirrhosis conditions and what diet one should eat to keep the liver functioning.

## Using Diet to Manage Decompensated Cirrhosis

The second stage of cirrhosis and a dangerous one is called decompensated cirrhosis. This is a condition where the liver is not able to perform all of its normal functions. As a result, patient may suffer from other severe conditions like fluid retention and mental confusion, known as encephalopathy.

For people suffering with decompensated cirrhosis, a high energy and high protein diet is recommended. To be more precise, you would need 35-40kcal and 1.5g of protein for every kg of your body weight per day. It is highly recommended that you must consult your certified doctor for further diet recommendations and treatment.

## Handling Fluid Retention

It has been found in the studies that some of the people, who have cirrhosis, may get a buildup of fluid in the stomach area. Other symptoms of this condition are swelling of the legs and feet. Due to the buildup of fluid in the stomach, one may feel bloated most of the times, but it is highly recommended that the person should drink enough fluids to avoid dehydration.

Cutting down on the amount of common salt in your food can help control fluid retention. The recommendation is to keep the salt content balanced, not too high and not too low. The anticipated amount of salt or sodium reduction in your diet is approx. 5.2g of salt per day.

The amount of salt in your own prepared food can be controlled but you may not control the salt contents in the foods that are available in the market. It is recommended that you always look at the labels on the food you buy. It will help you keep your salt intake in control.

The best place to look for this information is the nutrition information on the food label. You need to look for the amount of salt per 100g. A food can be called low in salt if the salt content is up to 0.3g salt or less per 100g or 0.1g sodium.

# Handling Hepatic Ecephalopathy

It has been found in the studies that some people with cirrhosis may develop poor memory and concentration conditions because the damaged liver is not in a position anymore to break the toxins from the bowel which then supposed to enter the bloodstream and carried to the brain.

Hepatic encephalopathy can also occur when a person with cirrhosis also has some other conditions such as diarrhea, dehydration, constipation, vomiting and infection or bleeding. In the past, people with hepatic encephalopathy were treated with a low protein diet but it has now been recognized that this was the wrong approach and that a high protein diet will help to improve the overall liver function. This applies to many internet sites as well that still wrongly suggest that a protein restricted diet is the solution for this condition.

If you are suffering with hepatic encephalopathy, you should:

- Aim to have four to six small meals per day that are rich in protein.
- Try to have a snack late in the evening that is high in carbs. This will aid in supporting your liver functions throughout night.
- Add poultry, eggs, fish and cheese to your diet as these are good alternatives to red meat as a source of protein.
- Add starchy foods such as potatoes, pasta, rice, cereals and pasta to your diet as these foods help in providing energy slowly over a longer period.

# CHAPTER 4:

# Various Types of Fatty Liver Conditions and Diets to Cure Them

## Liver failure

When you have liver failure, it means that your liver has lost most, if not all, of its liver function a serious condition that requires emergency medical attention. The first symptoms you are going to notice are diarrhea, extreme nausea, fatigue and a loss of appetite. Because these symptoms are common to many other ailments that your body could be suffering from, it can be really difficult to know that your liver is actually failing.

However as liver failure becomes more and more advanced, the symptoms continue advancing too and the patient may start getting very disoriented and confused and unusually sleepy. If unattended to, there is a very high risk of coma or in the worst-case scenario, death. Doctors will try to save any part of the liver that is still working and if this is impossible the other option will be a transplant.

In an event of a liver failure due to cirrhosis, it means that the patient's liver has been gradually getting sicker and failing over time, possibly for a number of years and is referred to as chronic liver failure or End Stage Liver Disease. Although very rare, liver failure could also be caused by malnutrition. Acute liver failure is when liver failure is very sudden, occurring in as little as two days and is usually cause by a medication overdose or a severe case of poisoning.

## Liver Cancer

Cancer that originates in the liver is referred to as primary liver cancer. Hepatitis B and cirrhosis are the two leading risk factors of primary liver cancer. However, it is important to note that cancer in the liver can progress at any stage of liver disease and that's why regular routine checkups are very important as they make it possible to catch cancer, if any, at a very early stage that's removable before it progresses to the entire liver.

## Alcoholic Liver Disease (ALD)

If you are a heavy drinker or have been drinking alcohol excessively, this is the first stage of injury to your liver due to buildup of fatty deposits. If proper care is taken and you stay away from alcohol, this can be completely reversed. As per the studies, only 20% of people with alcohol related fatty liver go on to develop inflammation (alcoholic hepatitis) and eventually cirrhosis.

People who have been drinking alcohol excessively and has alcoholic liver damage have been found most of the times malnourished or undernourished which means their body lacks in nutrients that it requires to function properly. This lack of nourishment could be due to several factors, some common ones are:

- If you are not eating well and just drinking, you are asking your body to work hard to process alcohol. Alcohol has no nutritional value but requires a lot of energy for the body to process it.
- Poor or un-balanced diet.
- Loss of appetite due to heavy drinking. If you are drinking as well as smoking, the condition will become worse. Smoking is known for suppressing hunger.
- Poor absorption of food nutrients as the liver is less able to produce bile to aid digestion.

You could be under nourished even if you are overweight. It all depends on what and how you eat. If you eat well and still becoming overweight, get yourself checked, if not already. This condition could be due to fluid retention.

You should be prescribed Vitamins B if you have been drinking excessively or at harmful levels. People with alcoholic liver disease generally lack the vitamin called thiamin, which is a vitamin B that helps the body to convert carbohydrates into energy. Consult your doctor or dietitian if this has not been prescribed.

## Acute Viral Hepatitis:

People who have an acute hepatitis, also known as short-term hepatitis, caused by a virus like hepatitis, should continue to eat a normal diet. In some cases, it is found that patients lose some weight in this condition. In a situation like this a patient may need extra nutrition to prevent unplanned weight loss. A high energy and high protein diet are recommended for such patients. A dietitian can advise on this.

## N.A.F.L.D - Non-Alcoholic Fatty Liver Disease

As the name suggests, non-alcoholic fatty liver disease is a condition when there is a fat buildup in the liver cells even if the patient does not drink alcohol excessively. At the initial stages, the fat deposits may not trigger any symptoms, but it has been found that in some cases, this may progress to inflammation called Nonalcoholic Steatohepatitis (NASH) which further can lead to scarring of the tissues in the liver and even cirrhosis.

People may still develop a fatty liver without excessive consumption of alcohol. There could be several factor or reasons of developing a fatty liver. Your likelihood of developing fatty liver conditions is higher if:

- Have diabetes.
- Are obese or overweight
- An insulin resistance body where your body does not respond to insulin as it should.
- Have high blood cholesterol.

You may be advised to make some changes to your diet and lifestyle, if you have been diagnosed with non-alcoholic fatty liver disease. These diet and lifestyle changes include:

- Eating a lot of vegetables and fruits.
- Eating slow-release starchy foods, such as potatoes and bread.
- Doing regular exercise such as walking, jogging or swimming.
- Reduce or stop the consumption of alcohol.
- Avoiding refined sugars and saturated fats which are commonly found in chocolate, cakes and biscuits.

It is also recommended to maintain a healthy weight for your age and build. If you have diabetes, it is suggested to work with your doctor to keep your blood sugar levels under good control. Consult your doctor if you have issues with high blood cholesterol levels or if you are insulin resistant.

## Chronic Viral Hepatitis

If you suffer from a long term hepatitis infection caused by a virus such as hepatitis B or hepatitis C and lasts for more than six to seven months, the condition is called a Chronic Viral Hepatitis. In such a condition, it is recommended to eat a normal well-balanced diet. Fasting due to any reasons is not recommended at all if you have chronic liver disease.

It is highly recommended to maintain an appropriate weight as per your height and build because it has been found in studies that more weight can increase and speed up the damages caused by hepatitis C and can slow down the recovery.

Some studies show that some people have conditions like poor appetite, nausea, vomiting and unintentional loss of weight during the treatment with anti-viral agents. If all or any of these conditions lasts for more than a few days, you must consult a doctor immediately.

## Autoimmune Hepatitis

Autoimmune hepatitis is also categorized as a chronic liver disease. It involves liver damage and inflammation due to an attack on the normal components and cells by the immune system. In a condition like this, sometimes, patients are prescribed steroids. In some cases, patients prescribed steroids find that their appetite increases over time and they gradually start gaining weight.

If you are suffering from autoimmune hepatitis and on steroids and have symptoms like increase in appetite and weight gain, it is still important and recommended to eat a well-balanced diet. If you are on steroids for a long time, it is important that you have been prescribed vitamin D and calcium by your doctor.

## Strategies to cut down on fat

If at all you need to cut down on the fat you eat, you also need to make sure that you avoid the hidden fats along with the ones you see in meat and greasy foods. The list below gives examples of high-fat foods and ideas for alternatives.

- Replace high fat containing butter, lard, margarine, mayonnaise and drippings with low fat alternatives.
- Replace full cream milk with semi skimmed or skimmed versions.
- Replace cheese with low fat hard cheese and low-fat cottage cheese.
- Reduce the intake of all kinds of cooking oil including olive oil, vegetable oil and sunflower oil. Use them in low amounts only. A good practice is to measure the amount you are adding using a tablespoon.
- *Stop eating fatty meats such as pork belly and duck*. You can replace these fatty meats with lean options like fish, poultry and lean red meat.
- *It is recommended to stop or reduce the amount of meat you eat.* Try to start eating more beans, vegetables, pulses and tofu.
- *It is good to stop eating fried chips, crisps and nuts.* You can replace these with oven baked chips or even completely replacing chips with a low-fat alternative such as jacket potato.
- *Replace cakes, pastry and biscuits with low-fat alternatives like scones*, teacakes and low-fat biscuits and cakes.
- *Stop the intake of processed foods*, as many processed foods are very high in fat content. Some of the examples are pizza, lasagna, ready-made curries etc. Try to replace these with a low-fat version, if possible and in small amounts only.
- *If you need to cut down the fat in your diet, you must ensure that you add and eat extra carbohydrates to compensate any descent in energy.* But you also need to understand that adding more carbohydrates means more starch and sugar, in your diet. It is recommended in this situation to take advice from a certified dietitian to make sure you are eating enough calories, protein and vitamins required by your body to function as needed.

## Strategies to cook with less fat

The following list provides some ideas on how to you can reduce the amount of fat you use in your cooking.

- Instead of frying, try Steaming, baking, boiling, steaming as your preferred method of cooking to avoid adding those extra fats.
- Skim fat off the surface of soups and casseroles.
- Always remove the skin from poultry before cooking such as chicken.
- Always trim down the visible fats off the meat.

## Strategies to deal with acidity

It has been found in some cases that people dealing with Primary biliary cirrhosis may have a bad acid taste in your mouth. They may also get heartburns which is a severe burning sensation in the chest. This burning sensation in chest and unpleasant acid taste in mouth is caused when the stomach acids escape into your food pipe.

In such a situation, it is recommended that you should try eating food in small quantities as much as possible. Eating food in little quantities may result in reducing stomach acids to escape into food pipe and causing burning sensations in the chest. As a best practice, try to carry small quantities of food with you all the time, just in case if you need to eat. Aim for foods high in carbs, such as plain biscuits, crackers, or breadsticks.

Another recommendation is to avoid heavy and big meals at night. Go with a small and healthy meal and include a snack for later time. You can also take an antacid after meals and before going to bed. Another trick to deal with this condition is to raise the head of your bed by five to six inches, if possible.

If none of the above-mentioned recommendations help and symptoms persist, discuss this with your doctor, who may recommend some other treatments.

## Food to eat and food to avoid

| Food to eat | Food to avoid | Food to reduce |
|---|---|---|
| Unsaturated Fats<br>Mushrooms<br>Fruits And Vegetables<br>Whole Grain Foods<br>Antioxidants<br>Dietary fiber<br>Cruciferous foods | Alcohol<br>Fried foods<br>Processed grains | Spices<br>High-sugar foods |

# CHAPTER 5:

# 21-Day Meal Plan

| WEEK 1 | Breakfast | Snack | Lunch | Dinner | Snack |
|--------|-----------|-------|-------|--------|-------|
| 1 | Superfood Muesli | Nut Cereal | Tasty Lime Cauliflower Rice | Quinoa Salad | Lime Pea Guacamole |
| 2 | Banana Oats | Salmon Stuffed Cucumbers | Tasty Lime Cauliflower Rice | Salmon with Tahini | Lemon Roasted Bell Pepper |
| 3 | Mini Frittatas | Triple C Shake | Tasty Lime Cauliflower Rice | Beef Curry | Strawberry Frozen Yogurt |
| 4 | The better Quiche Lorraine | Homemade Nutella | Steamed Chicken Salad | Lemon-Pepper tuna Bake | Carrot Chips |
| 5 | Easy Avocado Pancake | Honey Chili Nuts | Steamed Chicken Salad | Hot Pork Meatballs | Asparagus Frittata |
| 6 | Sauteed Mushrooms & Eggs | Carrot and Parsnip French Fries | Steamed Chicken Salad | Cheesy Keto Zucchini Soup | Coconut mango Lassi |
| 7 | Berry Oats | Carrot and Parsnip French Fries | Ultimate Liver Detox Soup | Steamed Chicken with Rainbow Salad Bowl | Trail Mix |

| WEEK 2 | Breakfast | Snack | Lunch | Dinner | Snack |
|---|---|---|---|---|---|
| 8 | Yogurt with Dates | Spiced Spinach Bites | Chicken and Carrot Soup | Steamed Chicken with Rainbow Salad Bowl | Spiced Toasted Almonds & Seed Mix |
| 9 | Vanilla Pancakes | Collard Green Tomatoes | Cauliflower Couscous Salad | Meatloaf | Banana Smoothie |
| 10 | Detox Porridge | Avocado Fudge | Chicken Quesadilla | Lemon Garlic Shrimp Zoodles | Orange Tarragon Chicken Salad Wrap |
| 11 | Savory Egg Gallettes | Oven Roasted Asparagus | Vegetarian Spanish Toast with Escalivada | Chicken & Veggies with Toasted Walnuts | Spiced Spinach Bites |
| 12 | Veggie Omelet | Almond Crackers | Ravaging Beef Pot Roast | Rosemary Citrus Shrimps | Spiced Spinach Bites |
| 13 | Pear Oatmeal | Spiced Toasted Almonds & Seed Mix | Pan-Seared Salmon Salad with Snow Peas & Grapefruit | Chicken and Carrot Stew | Oven Roasted Asparagus |
| 14 | Bacon Veggies Combo | Apple Chips | Avocado Tuna Salad | Detox Salad with Steamed White Fish | Cheesy Kale Chips |

| WEEK 2 | Breakfast | Snack | Lunch | Dinner | Snack |
|---|---|---|---|---|---|
| 15 | Beets Omelette | Chocolate Bread | Cauliflower Risotto | Mediterranean Sauteed Chicken | Roasted Asparagus |
| 16 | Omelette | Cardamom Tart | Turkey with Tomatoes | Chicken Stuffed with Cheese | Asparagus Frittata |
| 17 | Onion Omelette | Pear Tart | Lean Turkey Paprikash | Greek Lemony Chicken Skewers | Roasted Radishes |
| 18 | 74. Brocc oli Omelette | Peach Pecan Pie | Pollo Fajitas | Creole Spaghetti | Radish Hash Browns |
| 19 | Beets Omelette | Butterfinger Pie | Chunky Chicken Quesadilla | Honey Almond Chicken Tenders | Strawberry Frozen Yogurt |
| 20 | Breakfast Beans | Strawberry Pie | Chicken Fettuccine with Shiitake Mushrooms | Parsley Chicken with Potatoes | Walnut & Spiced Apple Tonic |
| 21 | Seeds and Lentils Oats | Pistachios Ice Cream | Chicken Yakitori | Baked Balsamic Fish | Basil & Walnut Pesto |

# CHAPTER 6:

# Shopping List

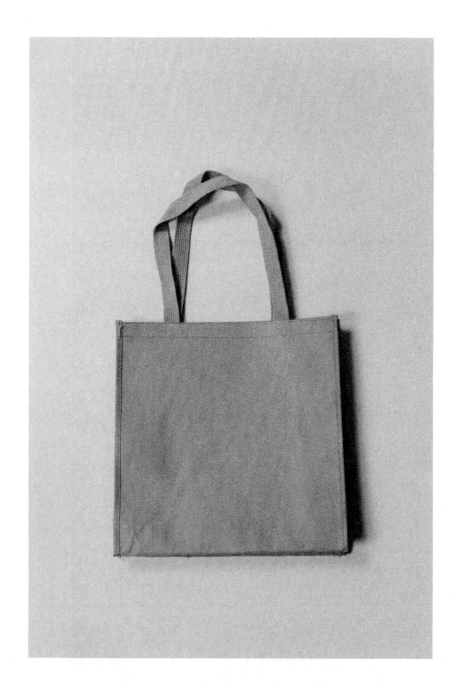

# Week 1

- Parsley
- Cherry Tomatoes
- Chorizo
- Cans Chickpeas
- Onion
- Dried Thyme
- Baby Bella Mushrooms
- Baby Potatoes
- Zucchini Or Summer Squash
- Campari Tomatoes
- Cup Olive Oil
- Lemon Juice
- Red Jalapeno
- Potatoes
- Sea Salt
- Soft Goat's Cheese
- Serrano Ham
- Chicken Broth
- Stale Bread
- Fresh Basil
- Mató Cheese
- Walnuts
- Eggplant
- Ciabatta
- Kosher Salt
- Banana
- Almond Milk
- Brewed Coffee
- Dates
- Cocoa Powder
- Chia Seeds
- Eggs
- Oregano, Dried
- Red Onion
- Baby Arugula
- Goat Cheese
- Spinach
- Green Apple
- Avocado,
- Coconut Water
- Parmesan, Grated
- Yellow Bell Pepper
- Red Bell Pepper
- Zucchini
- Olive Oil
- Chives,
- Berries
- Yogurt
- Red Pepper Flakes
- Cauliflower
- Cream Cheese
- Whipping Cream
- Wild Salmon
- Balsamic Vinegar
- Lamb Shoulder
- Chicken Breasts
- Chicken Thighs
- Powdered Stevia
- Cumin, Ground
- Salmon Fillets
- Can Red Salmon
- Fresh Horseradish
- Crackers,
- Whole Milk Greek Yogurt
- Ground Black Pepper
- Dijon Mustard
- Extra Virgin Olive Oil
- Fresh Tarragon
- Chicken
- Almonds
- Lettuce Leaves
- Avocado
- Red Bell Pepper
- Quinoa
- Mushrooms
- Feta
- Whole Wheat Flour
- Salt
- Garlic Yogurt Sauce
- Fresh Dill
- Lemon
- Berries
- Gelatin Powder
- Mozzarella Cheese
- Pepperoni
- Black Olives
- Ricotta Cheese
- Fresh Basil

- Cayenne
  Pepper

# Week 2

- Oats
- Milk
- Vanilla Extract
- Ground Cinnamon
- Honey
- Plain Yogurt
- Butter
- Yellow Onion
- Eggs
- Coconut Flakes
- Chili Pepper
- Cheddar Cheese
- Canola Oil
- Green Bell Pepper,
- Bacon
- Parmesan Cheese
- Mayonnaise
- Scallion
- Brown Rice
- Baby Arugula
- Canned Garbanzo Beans
- Feta Cheese
- Basil
- Lemon

- Lemon Zest
- Olive Oil
- Yeast
- Baking Powder
- Wheat Flour
- Butter
- Sugar
- White Onion
- Tomato
- Cucumber
- Fresh Cilantro
- Jalapeno Pepper
- Lime
- Corn Tortillas
- Canola Oil
- Cheddar Cheese
- White Beans
- Pitas
- Chicken Breast
- Red Onion
- Dried Oregano
- Greek Yogurt, Plain
- Plum Tomato
- Cucumber
- Fresh Dill
- Iceberg Lettuce

- Tahini Paste
- Pine Nuts
- Tomato Paste
- Walnuts
- Pecan Nuts
- Bird's-Eye Chili,
- Cauliflower Head
- Low-Fat Mozzarella Cheese,
- Italian Seasoning
- Grapes
- Sticks Of Celery
- Matcha Powder
- Vegetable Oil
- Red Pepper Flakes
- Zucchinis,
- Apples,
- White Sugar
- Carrots,
- Corn-Starch
- Maple Syrup
- Nutritional Yeast
- Kales

# Week 3

- Eggs
- Black Pepper
- Olive Oil
- Cheese
- Basil
- Beets
- Can Chickpeas,
- Can Fava Beans,
- Garlic
- Fresh Lemon Juice
- Cayenne
- Fresh Parsley
- Tomato,
- Radishes
- Extra-Virgin Olive Oil
- Red Lentils
- Pumpkin Seeds,
- Olive Oil
- Rolled Oats
- Coconut Flesh,
- Honey
- Orange Zest,
- Greek Yogurt
- Blackberries
- Chicken Breast
- Artichoke Hearts,
- Black Pepper
- Tomatoes, Sun-Dried
- Feta Cheese
- Leaf Parsley,
- Vegetable Broth

- Olive Oil
- Onions,
- Parmesan Cheese
- Cauliflower
- Turkey Breast Filets
- Olive Tapenade
- Egg Noodles
- Mushroom
- Onions
- Turkey
- Chicken Broth,
- Sweet Paprika
- Greek Yogurt
- Worcestershire Sauce
- Apple Cider Vinegar
- Soy Sauce With Less Sodium
- Chili Powder
- Dash Hot Sauce
- Skinless Chicken Breasts
- Wholewheat
- Lemon
- Wholewheat Fettuccine
- Boneless, Skinless Breasts Of Chicken,
- Garlic Cloves And Hazelnuts
- Shiitake Mushrooms

- Sherry Or White Wine To Prepare
- Low-Sodium Chicken Broth
- Ginger
- Scallions
- Ground Turkey
- Rubbed Wheat Germ
- Parmesan Cheese
- Black Chili Pepper
- Orange,
- Grapefruit,
- Pineapple
- Fresh Ginger
- Cucumbers
- Kale
- Beets
- Tangerine
- Lime
- Dandelion Greens
- Knob Ginger
- Spinach
- Kale Leaves
- Celery Stalks,
- Chia Seeds
- All-Purpose Flour
- Butter
- Shallots
- Dry Marsala Wine
- Heavy Cream
- Fresh Thyme

- Boneless, Skinless Chicken Breasts
- Orzo Pasta
- Pitas
- Greek Yogurt
- Garlic,

- Kalamata Olives
- Tatziki Sauce
- Garlic.
- Chicken
- Cinnamon Stick

- Berries
- Bay Leaf
- White Wine
- Fresh Thyme
- Fresh Basil
- Kalamata Olives

# CHAPTER 7:

# Advice And Guidance

## How to Eliminate Toxins from Your Liver for Better Health, Weight Loss, and Energy

As we have stated throughout the previous chapters, the liver is responsible for metabolizing fats, which unlike proteins and carbs, are very difficult to digest. It's therefore prudent to avoid excessive consumption of fats to avoid overworking your liver which can lead to fatty liver disease, as is the case with people suffering from obesity.

## Caution when taking medication:

Some medicinal combinations can be heavily taxing on your liver and it's always advisable that all medicine that you take is prescribed by a medical professional. Additionally, avoid mixing medication with natural remedies as this too can be overwhelming to your liver. It is especially important that you not mix alcohol with medicine as this can be too heavy on your liver to the point of liver failure. It is important that you ask your doctor if it's okay to consume alcohol with the drugs you have been prescribed for.

## Avoid excessive consumption of alcohol:

Heavy alcohol consumption leads to cirrhosis of the liver over time. The process of your liver breaking down alcohol involves the production of free radicals and chemicals such as acetaldehyde. For serious damage to occur in your liver, it takes about a liter of wine, or its equivalent on a daily basis for 20 years in women. For women, it takes less than half.

## Practice safe sex:

At the moment there is no vaccination for hepatitis C. As such you should practice caution when it comes to sex, piercings and tattoos.

## Avoid aerosol/ airborne chemicals:

When using gardening, housecleaning chemicals and paint, ensure that your environment is well ventilated and also put on a mask. Try as much as possible to reduce your inhalation of toxins as the liver is forced to process all toxins and this can cause liver problems especially if you are exposed to toxic agents on a regular basis.

## Get the necessary vaccinations:
It is important that you get vaccinated especially if you are intending on travelling to a place where malaria, Hepatitis A and B may be a concern. Yellow fever has been shown to lead to liver failure, malaria grows and multiplies in your liver. Take the necessary precautions by taking the recommended vaccines and drugs.

## Avoid exposure to foreign blood and germs:
If you come in contact with another person's blood you should for immediate medical attention. Also avoid sharing personal items such as needles and toothbrushes. Take care of yourself to avoid exposure to toxins.

weight loss? If this is something that is happening to you regularly, I have a few powerful alternative practices to recommend. These practices are a great way for many people to detoxify their livers without the use of harsh chemicals or other pharmaceuticals.

## Powerful alternative practices to detoxify your liver
The first practice should be reducing your consumption of hydrogenated oils and trans fats. These hydrogenated oils have been shown to cause liver damage and in some studies, they were even shown to block the production of essential fatty acids in people that were consuming them in their daily diets.

## Healthful oils to use instead of hydrogenated oils:
Avocados, walnuts, flaxseed oil, walnut oil, olive oil, macadamia nuts and butter made from butter. One avocado contains about 12.5 grams of fat which is about 3/4 of a tablespoon. If you eat one avocado a day you should be able to get enough essential fatty acids in your diet without having to take supplemental EPA and DHA.

## Time to detox:
I recommend around 5 days of cleansing. The first morning, I recommend an easy cleanse which involves 3 cups of lemon water and 1/2 cup of raspberry leaf tea made fresh with water and lemon juice. For the next 3 days, I like to eat as much as is comfortable for you. You can do as much or as little as you like, but my experience has been that people feel the most energetic after they have eaten a reasonable amount.

## Make it easy:
Please use organic produce whenever you can, especially if you have been consuming the hydrogenated oils and trans fats.

The second practice is reducing your consumption of artificial sweeteners. Since artificial sweeteners have been shown to cause heart disease and cancer in animal studies, I do not recommend them to my patients. If a person is a tea drinker or a coffee drinker, there are some alternatives that you can try.

Essential fatty acids are vital to liver function and when they're not available in the body, many health issues can occur. Essential fatty acids help with inflammation in the body, reduce cholesterol and triglyceride levels in the blood and also support healthy skin and hair. inflammation.

# CHAPTER 8:

# Powerful Alternative Practice to Detoxify Liver

It has been observed that people who are obese or overweight are less satiated after eating, resulting in an overeating tendency. It's important for us to not overeat. Fatty liver diet is not the best solution. A fatty liver diet doesn't work for everyone, especially if you have a lot of fat on your frame.

Water enriched with vitamin C is essential to keep the liver functioning properly, glasses of water also help to flush the liver.

It is also good for the body as well as the health of your liver as well as for people who have a fatty liver diet.

You should drink about three liters of water daily. But it's important to drink only clean water so you can hydrate yourself well and avoid problems from drinking too much toxic substances that are in tap water.

Drink lots of green tea. Although green tea contains caffeine, it is also abundant in antioxidants and polyphenols which boost your liver health and fights disease.

Eat more fruits and vegetables, which will not only help to remove toxins but will also deliver the vitamins and nutrients needed by the liver.

Eat fatty fish can be helpful as can omega-3s found in fish oils or supplements.

Avoid processed foods as they're usually high in nitrates and sodium which can be harmful to the liver

For those who are very overweight, the best thing you can do is to lose weight. If this is not an option, then you can follow a low-fat diet which doesn't include fatty foods.

Reducing your fructose intake may help as well as fiber, fiber and potassium rich foods and the right amounts of exercise and healthy lifestyle habits

Each person is unique in that they respond differently to diet and exercise, so you will need to pay close attention to how your body is reacting. Always remember that there is no one diet that will work for everyone!

Not everyone needs to follow a fatty liver diet, but it is important that you talk to your doctor about it first.

You should always consult with your doctor before or while following the fatty liver diet.

Obviously, the amount of water an individual needs is dependent on many factors such as weight, activity level, and environment. The general recommendation for most adults who are not exerting themselves outdoors in the heat is 8 cups per day.

Liver detox treatments can often appear, well, simplistic. But here, the simple truth is that water improves the liver move toxins out of its own cellular systems and run them on their path out of your body.

A great general rule of thumb is to aim for 4 liters of water per day. Break away from carbonated water or water in plastic drink containers.

## TWO Secret Liver Detox Practices That Even Hollywood Stars Use

### 1) Coffee edema detox *(From Gerson therapy)*

An enema is coffee enema is well known for its purifying properties, unlike classic enemas, it is prepared using water and coffee to take advantage of the benefits of caffeine.

The coffee enema was invented in 1917 as an alternative medicine method. It was brought to prominence by German-American physician Max Gerson, who gave the therapy its name. Gerson thought that coffee enemas were more useful than saline enemas for detoxifying the body and helping patients regain health, because it was able to pass through the intestines and reach the liver. In fact, coffee taken rectally is absorbed by the hemorrhoidal vein and rectal mucosa and within minutes is transported to the liver and gallbladder. At this point there is a strong release of bile, which is charged and carries away a large amount of metabolic waste and toxins, which through the last part of the intestine and the rectum are finally evacuated with the rest of the enema.

This is a powerful detox that allows the liver to get rid of a large amount of toxins and metabolic waste in a few minutes.

The effects in the short to medium term are: significant increase in energy and vitality in general, a sense of greater well-being, increased mental clarity, improved digestion, increased skin radiance, general detoxification of the whole body, and elimination of intestinal parasites.

### 2) liver flush- *(Andreas Moritz)*

Andreas Moritz in which the author illustrates the process of flushing and expelling gallstones that he developed and that can be done independently at home. This simple, inexpensive, painless and safe natural method of purification can help us improve our energy, free us from pain and give us beauty and mental clarity, opening the door to a disease-free life.

The actual washing consists of taking almost exclusively epsom salt, also known as English salt or bitter salt (chemically it is magnesium sulfate heptahydrate), cold-pressed extra virgin olive oil and grapefruit or orange extracts. This particular diet, combined with a few hours of rest (strictly on the stomach, with the head slightly elevated), would have the ability to promote the expulsion, through subsequent defecation, of a large number of gallstones, distinguishable by the green color and the fact that they float while everything else sinks.

Repeated at a distance of 2-3 weeks, the protocol would guarantee - according to its promoters - a "complete cleaning of the liver" and significant benefits for those who undergo it.

*Herbal teas could be an alternative option when it comes to keeping up your fluids.* Apart from that, they are easy to drink, can be enjoyed hot or cold, and benefit our health.

Before exploring the aisles and wide range of herbal teas available, it is best to read the package before purchasing. Do not buy any teas with added colorants, sugars, and flavors. Herbal tea should just be that, herbal.

As herbs go, they have been considered medicinal for centuries and can be self-prescribed to treat certain ailments.

Herbal teas constitute a good choice. Grab a break from inflammatory foods such as sugar, milk, gluten, caffeine, and alcohol. Limit your exposure to foods that are low in nutrients, such as chips, cookies, pastries, and muffins. Still, feel like you can go through a bag of cookies or chips, but still feel hungry? That's because the food is empty calories, and you don't get the best bang for your buck. Such hyper-palatable foods don't fill you up (yet you consume the high calories), so you might end up eating more than you need.

## herbs, leaves, roots and bud extracts.

*Nettle leaf:* Nettle is rich in silica, iron, and potassium and it is used for treating inflammation.

*St. Mary's thistle:* Thistle tea is known to restore the cells within the liver and protect it. It is also a novel herbal tea for treating headaches.

*Dandelion root:* Dandelion root stimulates your digestive system and cleans the body of any excess hormonal build-up, which may cause mood swings and low energy levels.

# CHAPTER 9:

# Bis - What is the proper physical activity for a healthy liver?

Regular exercise helps remove the body's toxins and shed fat. Subcutaneous fat (the fat you can pinch) contains toxins, and exercise may help shed the fat. Here are some of the ways the workout allows the body to detoxify: you sweat. The skin is cleansed by transpiration from the inside out. Many contaminants may be released by sweating through the skin. Moving the body forces heavier respiration, circulation, stretching, and sweating —all of which accelerate detoxification. Moving your body helps both blood and lymph circulate. The more they circulate, the more they can do the job of cleaning the liver and lymph nodes and purifying the blood and lymph. Exercise enhances bowel movement and digestion. Exercising stimulates the heart and helps increase the capacity of the lungs to remove carbon dioxide as a waste product.

When you can't fit into regular exercise, then walk often in your everyday life, at least. Wake up and walk around regularly, wake up against sitting too much, take the stairs, park farther out, do chores vigorously, walk the dog. Anything that pushes the body is better than being sedentary.

There are many types of exercise you can undertake. Broadly speaking, these fall into gym oriented or non-gym-oriented exercises.

If you have to go to a place, say your office, instead of taking the bus or car or train, walk to the place if the distance is walk worthy. You need to be practical too, you cannot walk 5 miles to go to the office.

If you enjoy outdoors, try cycling, it will tone up every muscle in the body. Swimming is another great option.

Joining the gym is not always essential. You can find many sources of good exercise in your everyday activities at home or at office.

## Running/Swimming/Sports

Low impact refers to the force your joints have to bear when carrying out the activity. Given that swimming happens in water, your joints bear minimal impact. The downside is that swimming happens to be extremely technical and it's a good idea to hire someone to teach you to swim in case you don't know how.

When starting off with these activities, it pays to start off slow and then slowly build your competence at them. Much like lifters increase the weight per session by five pounds, you can try to carry out the activity or five more minutes per session.

This is because the physical movement you undertake will build your strength up to a certain level and to progress further, you will need to perform greater amounts of that activity or go to the gym and work on increasing your strength.

Therefore, it pays to go to the gym and work on your strength. Your performance in other areas will increase as well. Lastly, physical activity levels you'll undertake by going to the gym and playing a sport will increase your metabolism and your body will become more efficient at burning whatever you fuel it with.

## Walking/Jogging

This exercise is for the females who have led an inactive lifestyle. You can start with a thirty minutes' walk in the park or even your home. Gradually increase it to forty-five minutes if possible. The walking is an amazing exercise if practiced daily. It is also the most basic form of exercise, leading females into a sense of activity. Interestingly, it is also preferred by women who were once very active but now have gone inactive physically. The best thing about walking is that it can be done in your own street or even rooftop.

An advanced form of walking is jogging. You can try it out in park. When you will start with walking and then gradually move towards jogging, there are a lot of benefits you will reap. Not only will your physical body be more active, but your mental health will also benefit from it.

## Light Aerobics

You haven't got much time? Or perhaps walking across the street or park is not possible? Light aerobics might just be what you need. You can start with light aerobics or low impact aerobics. There are a lot of YouTube videos available online. You can take a start from there. You will only need to do these 20 minutes a day for three to four days per week. All you need is a laptop to watch its video from and an empty space like a room. Don't exert too much pressure on your body. The fellows in the videos are experts. You just have to do the exercise and move your body.

## Stretching/Yoga

The stretching exercises are naturally the best ones. You can easily do the yoga for adults on everyday basis. The best results come when you pair it with light aerobics or walking. Yoga or stretching exercises have immense benefits. They relieve joint pain, provide your bones strength and flexibility, and increase your immunity. The stretching exercises also allow your body to be more flexible and stronger. Other than that, your mind will be relaxed as your body does the stretching

The same rule with light aerobics goes here too. You will need to take it easy and slow. Only stretch your body till a mild discomfort. Don't push too hard.

Yoga routine is easily available. Naturally, the best duo I have seen in some females was doing mild yoga in morning and pairing it with light aerobics or walking in the evening.

## Balance

There are plenty of light exercises that focus on improving your balance. Naturally, some poses of yoga also focus on balance. It is somewhat a crucial part of your health. You should focus on it quite often.

## Gym Work

Broadly speaking, there are two activities everyone carries out in the gym. They either hit the weights (or train for strength and shape) or perform cardio. Cardio and strength are two ends of a scale and it is physically impossible for human beings to have elite cardio levels and strength levels at the same time.

The intensity of your workouts is what determines this. For the average person, working out for strength and then performing some form of cardio for close to ten or fifteen minutes is more than enough to achieve a balance. Your objective should be to train for strength and perform cardio at the end of it.

## Cardio Programs

All cardio programs fall into two broad types: Anaerobic and aerobic. The former refers to when you train on an oxygen deficit and the latter is when you have a steady supply of oxygen. Anaerobic exercise is shorter in duration since there's only so long, we can function without oxygen.

Strength training and weightlifting take care of the anaerobic portion of cardio pretty well. Once you start lifting heavier weights as the program dictates, you'll train this side of your cardiovascular system. As for the aerobic side, activities such as running, and swimming do a great job of training this. Cycling is another activity that you can undertake.

You have two choices when it comes to timing your cardio routine. You can either perform it on alternate days with strength training or you can add a session at the end of it. Alternatively, you can sprinkle in the odd day of sports or cardio training during the week along with performing it at the end of your workout session.

The biggest reason for this has to do with resting. Many beginners to exercise underestimate the importance of rest. Real progress isn't made in the gym. It is made when you sleep. This is when your body repairs itself and gets stronger.

You'll find that after a tough workout session, you'll need to sleep for longer periods of time. Your body will adjust over time, and you'll find that eight hours will be enough. However, if you were to alternate your cardio and strength days, you'll overwork yourself and are less likely to stick to a regimen. One of the biggest benefits of a program like Starting Strength is that you'll workout for just three days a week. This is because you'll be performing compound lifts that take a lot out of you. In other words, you have four days of the week left to do whatever you wish instead of being stuck in the gym. Why would you want to reduce this time by performing extended cardio sessions?

Vary your choice of cardio after your workouts. Swim one day, cycle the next, run on the third and so on. The elliptical machine in the gym is also a great choice. If you find yourself exhausted, then feel free to skip cardio altogether. Strength training by itself will bring your cardio capacity up to a good level.

# HIIT

HIIT stands for High Intensity Interval Training. This is how it works: You perform an activity extremely fast for a short period, say for half a minute, rest for 20 seconds, and then get back to performing the activity for half a minute again. You repeat this for close to ten to fifteen minutes.

The fact is that HIIT is a great way to lose fat. Perform HIIT while fasted and the fat will practically melt right off. The downside of HIIT is that it can cause muscle loss since you'll have to exert so much more effort.

You need to have a certain strength level before HIIT makes sense for you to implement. Also, don't think of HIIT as being a workout by itself. Some practitioners choose to portray it this way but HIIT will build your strength to a certain level beyond which you'll need to resort to weights to make progress.

# CHAPTER 10:

# Breakfast Recipes

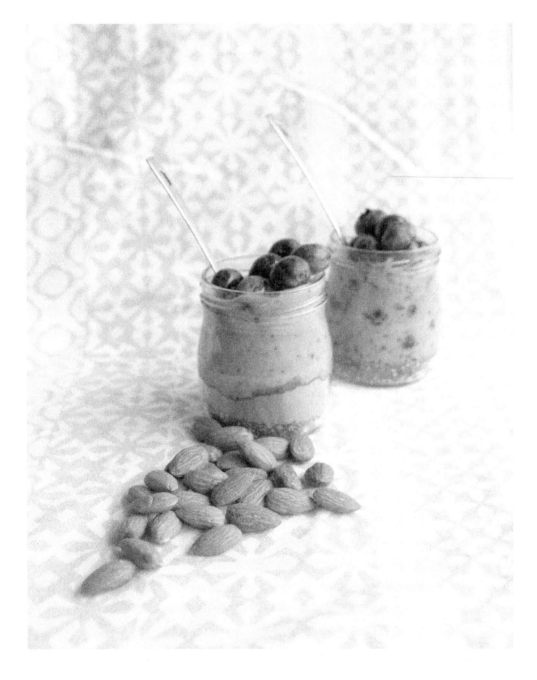

## 1. Banana Oats
**Preparation Time: 15 Minutes**
**Cooking Time:** 0
**Servings:** 2
**Ingredients:**
1 banana, peeled and sliced
3/4 cup almond milk
1/2 cup cold brewed coffee
2 dates, pitted
2 tablespoons cocoa powder
1 cup rolled oats
1 and 1/2 tablespoons chia seeds
**Directions:**
In a blender, combine the banana with the milk and the rest of the ingredients, pulse, divide into bowls and serve for breakfast.
**Nutrition:**
Calories 451
Fat 25.1
Fiber 9.9
Carbs 55.4
Protein 9.3

## 2. Slow cooked Peppers Frittata
**Preparation Time:** 10 Minutes
**Cooking Time:** 3 hours
**Servings:** 3
**Ingredients:**
1/2 cup almond milk
8 eggs, whisked
Salt and black pepper to the taste
1 teaspoon oregano, dried
1 and 1/2 cups roasted peppers, chopped
1/2 cup red onion, chopped
4 cups baby arugula
1 cup goat cheese, crumbled
Cooking spray
**Directions:**
In a bowl, combine the eggs with salt, pepper and the oregano and whisk.

Grease your slow cooker with the cooking spray, arrange the peppers and the remaining ingredients inside and pour the eggs mixture over them.
Put the lid on and cook on Low for 3 hours.
Divide the frittata between plates and serve.
**Nutrition:**
Calories 259
Fat 20.2
Fiber 1
Carbs 4.4
Protein 16.3

## 3. Avocado and Apple Smoothie
**Preparation Time:** 10 Minutes
**Cooking Time:** 0
**Servings:** 3
**Ingredients:**
3 cups spinach
1 green apple, cored and chopped
1 avocado, peeled, pitted and chopped
3 tablespoons chia seeds
1 teaspoon honey
1 banana, frozen and peeled
2 cups coconut water
**Directions:**
In your blender, combine the spinach with the apple and the rest of the ingredients, pulse, divide into glasses and serve
**Nutrition:**
Calories 168 Fat 10.1
Fiber 6 Carbs 21
Protein 2.1

## 4. Mini Frittatas
**Preparation Time: 15** Minutes
**Cooking Time: 15** Minutes
**Servings:** 3
**Ingredients:**
1 yellow onion, chopped
1 cup parmesan, grated

1 yellow bell pepper, chopped
1 red bell pepper, chopped
1 zucchini, chopped
Salt and black pepper to the taste
8 eggs, whisked
A drizzle of olive oil
2 tablespoons chives, chopped

**Directions:**

Heat up a pan with the oil over medium high heat, add the onion, the zucchini and the rest of the ingredients except the eggs and chives and sauté for 5 minutes stirring often.

Divide this mix on the bottom of a muffin pan, pour the eggs mixture on top, sprinkle salt, pepper and the chives and bake at 350 degrees F for 10 minutes.

Serve the mini frittatas for breakfast right away.

**Nutrition:**

Calories 55
Fat 3
Fiber 0.7
Carbs 3.2
Protein 4.2

## 5. Berry Oats

**Preparation Time:** 8 Minutes
**Cooking Time:** 0
**Servings:** 1
**Ingredients:**

1/2 cup rolled oats
1 cup almond milk
1/4 cup chia seeds
A pinch of cinnamon powder
2 teaspoons honey
1 cup berries, pureed
1 tablespoon yogurt

**Directions:**

In a bowl, combine the oats with the milk and the rest of the ingredients except the yogurt, toss, divide into bowls, top with the yogurt and serve cold for breakfast.

**Nutrition:**

Calories 420
Fat 30.3
Fiber 7.2
Carbs 35.3
Protein 6.4

## 6. Sundried Tomatoes Oatmeal

**Preparation Time:** 15 Minutes
**Cooking Time:** 25 Minutes
**Servings:** 4
**Ingredients:**

3 cups water
1 cup almond milk
1 tablespoon olive oil
1 cup steelcut oats
1/4 cup sundried tomatoes, chopped
A pinch of red pepper flakes

**Directions:**

In a pan, mix the water with the milk, bring to a boil over medium heat.

Meanwhile, heat up a pan with the oil over mediumhigh heat, add the oats, cook them for about 2 minutes and transfer m to the pan with the milk.

Stir the oats, add the tomatoes and simmer over medium heat for 23 minutes.

Divide the mix into bowls, sprinkle the red pepper flakes on top and serve for breakfast.

**Nutrition:**

Calories 170
Fat 17.8
Fiber 1.5
Carbs 3.8
Protein 1.5

## 7. Quinoa Muffins

**Preparation Time:** 15 Minutes
**Cooking Time:** 30 Minutes
**Servings:** 6
**Ingredients:**

1 cup quinoa, cooked

6 eggs, whisked
Salt and black pepper to the taste
1 cup Swiss cheese, grated
1 small yellow onion, chopped
1 cup white mushrooms, sliced
1/2 cup sundried tomatoes, chopped
**Directions:**
In a bowl, combine the eggs with salt, pepper and the rest of the ingredients and whisk well.
Divide this into a silicone muffin pan, bake at 350 degrees F for 30 minutes and serve for breakfast.
**Nutrition:**
Calories 123
Fat 5.6
Fiber 1.3
Carbs 10.8
Protein 7.5

## 8. Cheese & Cauliflower Bake

**Preparation Time:** 15 Minutes
**Cooking Time:** 4 hours
**Servings:** 2
**Ingredients:**
1 head cauliflower, cut into florets
1/2 cup cream cheese
1/4 cup whipping cream
2 Tablespoons lard (or butter, if you prefer)
1 Tablespoon lard (or butter, if you prefer) to grease the crockpot
1 teaspoon salt
1/2 teaspoon fresh ground black pepper
1/2 cup yellow cheese, Cheddar, shredded
6 slices of bacon, crisped and crumbled
**Directions:**
Grease the crockpot.
Add all the ingredients, except the cheese and the bacon.
Cook on low for 3 hours.

Open the lid and add cheese. Recover, cook for an additional hour.
Top with the bacon and serve.
**Nutrition:**
Calories: 278
Fat: 15g
Net Carbohydrates: 3g
Protein: 32g
Fiber: 1g
Net Carbs: 2g

## 9. Ham & Cheese Broccoli Brunch Bowl

**Preparation Time: 15 Minutes**
**Cooking Time:** 8 hours
**Servings:** 4
**Ingredients:**
1 medium head of broccoli, chopped small
4 cups vegetable broth
2 Tablespoons olive oil
1 teaspoon mustard seeds, ground
3garlic cloves, minced
Salt and pepper to taste
2 cups Cheddar cheese, shredded
2 cups ham, cubed
Pinch of paprika
**Directions:**
Add all ingredients to the crockpot in order of the list.
Cover, cook on low for 8 hours.
**Nutrition:**
Calories: 690 Fat: 48g
Carbohydrates: 16g
Protein: 40g Fiber: 3g
Net Carbohydrates: 13g

## 10. Zucchini & Spinach with Bacon

**Preparation Time: 15** Minutes
**Cooking Time:** 6 hours
**Servings:** 4
**Ingredients:**
8 slices bacon
1 Tablespoon olive oil

4 medium zucchinis, cubed
2 cups baby spinach
1 red onion, diced
6garlic cloves, sliced thin
1 cup chicken broth
Salt and pepper to taste
**Directions:**
In a pan, heat the olive oil, brown the bacon for 5 minutes. Break it into pieces in the pan. Place remaining ingredients in crockpot, pour the bacon and fat from the pan over the ingredients.
Cover, cook on low for 6 hours.
**Nutrition:**
Calories: 171 Fat: 16g
Net Carbohydrates: 6g
Protein: 2g Fiber: 2g   Carbohydrates: 8g

## 11. The Better Quiche Lorraine

**Preparation Time: 15** Minutes
**Cooking Time:** 4 hours
**Servings: 3**
**Ingredients:**
1 Tablespoon butter
10 eggs, beaten
1 cup heavy cream
1 cup Cheddar cheese, shredded
Pinch fresh ground black pepper
10 strips of bacon, crisped and crumbled
1/2 cup fresh spinach, chopped
**Directions:**
Butter the crockpot.  In a large bowl, mix all the ingredients, except bacon crumbles.   Transfer mixture to the crockpot, sprinkle bacon on top.
Cover, cook on low for 4 hours. (In the last 15 minutes' watch carefully, not to overcook it.)
**Nutrition:**
Calories: 260
Fat: 21g Net Carbohydrates: 4g

Protein: 14g Fiber: 1g
Carbohydrates: 5g

## 12. Spinach & Sausage Pizza

**Preparation Time: 15 Minutes**
**Cooking Time:** 25 Minutes
**Servings: 3**
**Ingredients:**
1 Tablespoon olive oil
1 cup lean ground beef
2 cups spicy pork sausage
2garlic cloves, minced
1 Tablespoon dry, fried onions
Salt and pepper to taste
1 3/4 cups sugarless readymade pizza sauce
3 cups fresh spinach
1/2 cup sliced pepperoni
1/4 cup pitted black olives, sliced
1/4 cup sundried tomatoes, chopped
1/2 cup spring onions, chopped
3 cups shredded mozzarella
**Directions:**
In a pan, heat the olive oil. Brown the beef, then the pork. Drain the oil off both portions of meat, mix together.
Pour the meat in the crockpot. Spread evenly and press down.
Alternate in layers: pizza sauce, toppings, and cheese.
Cover and cook on low for 25 Minutes.

**Nutrition:**
Calories: 259
Fat: 13g
Carbohydrates: 5g
Protein: 16g Fiber: 2g
Net Carbohydrates: 7g

## 13. Three Cheese Artichoke Hearts Bake

**Preparation Time: 15 Minutes**
**Cooking Time:** 2 hours
**Servings: 3**
**Ingredients:**

1 cup Cheddar cheese, grated
1/2 cup dry Parmesan cheese
1 cup cream cheese
1 cup spinach, chopped
1 clove of garlic, crushed
1 jar artichoke hearts, chopped
Salt and pepper to taste

**Directions:**
Place all the ingredients in the crockpot. Mix lightly.
Cover, cook on high for 2 hours.

**Nutrition:**
Calories: 141
Fat: 11.5g
Carbohydrates: 0.6g
Protein: 8.9g
Fiber: 0g
Net Carbohydrates: 0.5g

## 14. SunDried Tomatoes Salad

**Preparation Time:** 10 Minutes
**Cooking Time:** 0
**Servings: 3**
**Ingredients:**
1 cup sundried tomatoes, chopped
4 eggs, hardboiled, peeled, and chopped
1/2 cup olives, pitted, chopped
1 small red onion, finely chopped
1/2 cup Greek yogurt
1 teaspoon lemon juice
1 teaspoon Italian seasonings

**Directions:**
In the salad bowl, mix up all ingredients and shake well.

**Nutrition:**
Calories: 120
Protein: 8.8g
Carbohydrates: 5.9g
Fat: 7.1g
Fiber: 1.5g

## 15. Greek Bowl

**Preparation Time:** 20 Minutes
**Cooking Time:** 7 Minutes
**Servings: 3**
**Ingredients:**
1/4 cup Greek yogurt
12 eggs
1/4 teaspoon ground black pepper
1/2 teaspoon salt
1 tablespoon avocado oil
1 cup cherry tomatoes, chopped
1 cup quinoa, cooked
1 cup fresh cilantro, chopped
1 red onion, sliced

**Directions:**
Boil the eggs in the water within 7 minutes. Then cool them in the cold water and peel.
Chop the eggs roughly and put them in the salad bowl.
Add Greek yogurt, ground black pepper, salt, avocado oil, tomatoes, quinoa, cilantro, and red onion.
Shake the mixture well. Serve.

**Nutrition:**
Calories: 253
Protein: 16.2g
Carbohydrates: 22.4g
Fat: 11g
Fiber: 2.9g

## 16. Morning Oats

**Preparation Time:** 20 Minutes
**Cooking Time:** 0
**Servings: 1**
**Ingredients:**
1 oz. pecans, chopped
1/4 cup oats
1/2 cup plain yogurt
1 date, chopped
1/2 teaspoon vanilla extract

**Directions:**
Mix up all ingredients and leave for 5 minutes.
Then transfer the meal to the serving bowls.

**Nutrition:**
Calories: 196

Protein: 6.5g
Carbohydrates: 16.5g
Fat: 11.6g
Fiber: 2.9g

## 17. Yogurt with Dates
**Preparation Time:** 15 Minutes
**Cooking Time:** 0
**Servings:** 3
**Ingredients:**
5 dates, pitted, chopped
2 cups plain yogurt
1/2 teaspoon vanilla extract
4 pecans, chopped
**Directions:**
Mix up all ingredients in the blender and blend until smooth.
Pour it into the serving cups.
**Nutrition:**
Calories: 215
Protein: 8.7g
Carbohydrates: 18.5g
Fat: 11.5g
Fiber: 2.3g

## 18. Baked Eggs with Parsley
**Preparation Time:** 20 Minutes
**Cooking Time:** 20 Minutes
**Servings:** 3
**Ingredients:**
2green bell peppers, chopped
3 tablespoons olive oil
1 yellow onion, chopped
1 teaspoon sweet paprika
6 tomatoes, chopped
6 eggs
1/4 cup parsley, chopped
**Directions:**
Warm a pan with the oil over medium heat, add all ingredients except eggs and roast them for 5 minutes.
Stir the vegetables well and crack the eggs.

Transfer the pan with eggs in the preheated to 360°F oven and bake them for 15 minutes.
**Nutrition:**
Calories: 167 Protein: .3g
Carbohydrates: 10.2g Fat: 11.8g
Fiber: 2.6g

## 19. Mushroom Casserole
**Preparation Time:** 15 Minutes
**Cooking Time:** 60 Minutes
**Servings:** 2
**Ingredients:**
2 eggs, beaten
1 cup mushrooms, sliced
2 shallots, chopped
1 teaspoon marjoram, dried
1/2 cup artichoke hearts, chopped
3 oz. Cheddar cheese, shredded
1/2 cup plain yogurt
**Directions:**
Mix up all ingredients in the casserole mold and cover it with foil.
Bake the casserole for 60 minutes at 355°F.
**Nutrition:**
Calories: 156
Protein: 11.2g
Carbohydrates: 6.2g
Fat: 9.7g
Fiber: 1.3g

## 20. Vanilla Pancakes
**Preparation Time:** 20 Minutes
**Cooking Time:** 2 Minutes
**Servings:** 5
**Ingredients:**
6 ounces' plain yogurt
1/2 cup wholegrain flour
1 egg, beaten
1 teaspoon vanilla extract
1 teaspoon baking powder
**Directions:**
Heat nonstick skillet well. Meanwhile, mix up all ingredients.

Pour the mixture into the skillet in the shape of the pancakes. Cook them for 1 minute per side. Serve.

**Nutrition:**
Calories: 202
Protein: 11.7g
Carbohydrates: 29.4g
Fat: 3.8g Fiber: 3.7g

## 21. Savory Egg Galettes

**Preparation Time:** 25 Minutes
**Cooking Time:** 25 Minutes
**Servings: 3**
**Ingredients:**
1/4 cup white onion, diced
1/4 cup bell pepper, chopped
1/2 teaspoon salt
1 teaspoon chili flakes
2 tablespoons olive oil
1 teaspoon dried dill
6 eggs, beaten
2 tablespoons plain yogurt
**Directions:**
Mix up onion, bell pepper, salt, and chili flakes in the pan. Add olive oil and dried dill. Sauté the ingredients for 5 minutes.

Then pour the beaten eggs into the square baking mold. Add sautéed onion mixture and plain yogurt.

Flatten the mixture and bake in the preheated to 360°F oven for 20 minutes. Cut the meal into galettes. Serve.

**Nutrition:**
Calories: 166 Protein: 9g
Carbohydrates: 2.4g Fat: 13.5g
Fiber: 0.3g

## 22. Walnuts Yogurt Mix

**Preparation Time: 15 Minutes**
**Cooking Time:** 2
**Servings: 3**
**Ingredients:**
2 and 1/2 cups Greek yogurt

1 and 1/2 cups walnuts, chopped
1 teaspoon vanilla extract
3/4 cup honey
2 teaspoons cinnamon powder
**Directions:**
In a bowl, combine the yogurt with the walnuts and the rest of the ingredients, toss, divide into smaller bowls and keep in the fridge for 10 minutes before serving for breakfast.

**Nutrition:**
calories 388
fat 24.6
fiber 2.9
carbs 39.1
protein 10.2

## 23. Spiced Chickpeas Bowls

**Preparation Time:** 10 Minutes
**Cooking Time:** 30 Minutes
**Servings: 3**
**Ingredients:**
15 ounces canned chickpeas, drained and rinsed
1/4 teaspoon cardamom, ground
1/2 teaspoon cinnamon powder
1 and 1/2 teaspoons turmeric powder
1 teaspoon coriander, ground
1 tablespoon olive oil
A pinch of salt and black pepper
3/4 cup Greek yogurt
1/2 cup green olives, pitted and halved
1/2 cup cherry tomatoes, halved
1 cucumber, sliced
**Directions:**
Spread the chickpeas on a lined baking sheet, add the cardamom, cinnamon, turmeric, coriander, the oil, salt and pepper, toss and bake at 375 degrees F for 30 minutes.

In a bowl, combine the roasted chickpeas with the rest of the ingredients, toss and serve for breakfast.

**Nutrition:**
calories 519 fat 34.5
fiber 13.3 carbs 49.8 protein 12

## 24. Orzo And Veggie Bowls
**Preparation time: 10 minutes**
**Cooking time: 0 minutes**
**Servings: 4**
**Ingredients:**
2 and 1/2 cups whole-wheat orzo, cooked
14 ounces canned cannellini beans, drained and rinsed
1 yellow bell pepper, cubed
1 green bell pepper, cubed
A pinch of salt and black pepper
3 tomatoes, cubed
1 red onion, chopped
1 cup mint, chopped
2 cups feta cheese, crumbled
2 tablespoons olive oil
1/4 cup lemon juice
1 tablespoon lemon zest, grated
1 cucumber, cubed
1 and 1/4 cup kalamata olives, pitted and sliced
3 garlic cloves, minced
**Directions:**
In a salad bowl, combine the orzo with the beans, bell peppers and the rest of the ingredients, toss, divide the mix between plates and serve for breakfast.
**Nutrition:**
calories 411
fat 17fiber 13
carbs 51protein 14

## 25. Green Beans with Toasted Almonds
**Preparation Time: 15 Minutes**
**Cooking Time: 81 Minutes**
**Servings: 3**
**Ingredients:**
1 1/2 pounds green beans, shredded
1/2 cup. finely toasted diced almonds

11/2 cups. pomegranate arils
4 tbsp. olive oil
Kosher salt and black pepper
**Directions:**
Boil green beans within salted water just until bite tender, about 81minutes. Then drain them inside a colander and transfer them to a medium bowl having cold water.
After 10minutes, drain well and put aside.
Inside another small size bowl, whisk together oil, kosher salt, and black pepper. Add the seasoned oil to the cooked beans, whisk to coat.
Organize the beans over a plate, then scatter diced almonds with pomegranate arils over the top.
**Nutrition:**
Calories: 421 Fat: 11g
Protein: 15g Carbs: 67g
Fiber: 11g
Sodium: 641mg

## 26. Mediterranean Avocado Salad
**Preparation Time: 15 Minutes**
**Cooking Time: 35 Minutes**
**Servings: 3**
**Ingredients:**
2 avocados, chopped and pitted
4 1/2oz. halloumi cheese, sliced into small cubes
2 Roma tomatoes, chopped
1/2 cucumber, chopped
1 shallot, diced
11/2 cups. pitted Kalamata olives
Olive oil, as required
16 basil leaves, minced
For Vinaigrette:
1 garlic clove, chopped
1 lemon, zested also juiced
11/2 cups. olive oil
1 1/2 tsp. Za'atar
Kosher salt and black pepper ?

**Directions:**

Make the vinaigrette. Put vinaigrette items inside a medium size can seal tightly then shake just until wellcombined. Place aside.

Inside a salad bowl, include the salad items leaving Halloumi also basil. Add the vinaigrette; combine well. Check then adjust seasoning, add additional Za'atar spice (if liked). Add minced basil, then toss well.

Add halloumi cheese. Mix the cubes with 1 1/2 tbsp. of oil inside a small size bowl; whisk well—warm a griddle on medium flame. Include the cheese cubes, then Steam for about 35minutes while flipping once from each side until finely browned.

Include the Halloumi within the salad. Serve right away

**Nutrition:**
Calories 213
Fat 17.3 g
Carbohydrates 9.5 g
Sugar 4.5 g
Protein 7.4 g
Cholesterol 9 mg

## 27. Braised Artichokes in Tomato Sauce

**Preparation Time:** 20 Minutes
**Cooking Time:** 2 hours
**Servings: 3**
**Ingredients:**
6 artichokes, cleaned
15oz. can of diced tomatoes
4 garlic cloves, chopped
1/3 cup. extra virgin olive oil
11/2 cups. dry white wine
1/2 tsp. red chili flakes
Kosher salt and Black pepper
1/2 cup. diced parsley
**Directions:**

Chop the artichokes in half, lengthwise. Inside a heavy casserole, warm the oil on medium flame.

Add garlic with pepper flakes, then fry for 60seconds.

Add white wine with tomatoes, including half the parsley.

Sprinkle with kosher salt and black pepper, then start boiling.

Include the artichokes chopside down; decrease the flame.

Simmer for 120 minutes while flipping artichokes halfway just until forktender also the sauce thickens. Whisk in the rest of the parsley, then move to a serving dish.

Scoop the sauce on the artichokes.

**Nutrition:**
Calories: 310
Fat: 16g
Protein: 10g
Carbs: 33g
 Fiber: 6g
Sodium: 243mg

## 28. Vanilla Oats

**Preparation time: 10 minutes**
**Cooking time: 10 minutes**
**Servings: 4**
**Ingredients:**
1/2 cup rolled oats
1 cup milk
1 teaspoon vanilla extract
1 teaspoon ground cinnamon
2 teaspoon honey
2 tablespoons Plain yogurt
1 teaspoon butter
**Directions:**
Pour milk in the saucepan and bring it to boil.

Add rolled oats and stir well.

Close the lid and simmer the oats for 5 minutes over the medium heat. The cooked oats will absorb all milk.

Then add butter and stir the oats well.

In the separated bowl, whisk together Plain yogurt with honey, cinnamon, and vanilla extract.

Transfer the cooked oats in the serving bowls.

Top the oats with the yogurt mixture in the shape of the wheel.

**Nutrition:**
calories 243
fat 20.2
fiber 1
carbs 2.8
protein 13.3

## 29. Mushroom-egg Casserole

**Preparation time: 10 minutes**
**Cooking time: 25 minutes**
**Servings: 3**
**Ingredients:**
1/2 cup mushrooms, chopped
1/2 yellow onion, diced
4 eggs, beaten
1 tablespoon coconut flakes
1/2 teaspoon chili pepper
1 oz Cheddar cheese, shredded
1 teaspoon canola oil
**Directions:**
Pour canola oil in the skillet and preheat well.

Add mushrooms and onion and roast for 5-8 minutes or until the vegetables are light brown.

Transfer the cooked vegetables in the casserole mold.

Add coconut flakes, chili pepper, and Cheddar cheese.

Then add eggs and stir well.

Bake the casserole for 15 minutes at 360F.

**Nutrition:**
Calories 152, fat 11.1, fiber 0.7, carbs 3, protein 10.4

## 30. Bacon Veggies Combo

**Preparation time: 10 minutes**

**Cooking time: 35 minutes**
**Servings: 4**
**Ingredients:**
1/2 green bell pepper, seeded and chopped
2 bacon slices
1/4 cup Parmesan Cheese
1/2 tablespoon mayonnaise
1 scallion, chopped
**Directions:**
Preheat the oven to 375 degrees F and grease a baking dish.

Place bacon slices on the baking dish and top with mayonnaise, bell peppers, scallions and Parmesan Cheese.

Transfer in the oven and bake for about 25 minutes.

Dish out to serve immediately or refrigerate for about 2 days wrapped in a plastic sheet for meal preparation ping.

**Nutrition:**
Calories: 197 Fat: 13.8g
Carbohydrates: 4.7gProtein: 14.3g
Sugar: 1.9g Sodium: 662mg

## 31. Brown Rice Salad

**Preparation time: 10 minutes**
**Cooking time: 0 minutes**
**Servings: 4**
**Ingredients:**
9 ounces brown rice, cooked
7 cups baby arugula
15 ounces canned garbanzo beans, drained and rinsed
4 ounces feta cheese, crumbled
3/4 cup basil, chopped
A pinch of salt and black pepper
2 tablespoons lemon juice
1/4 teaspoon lemon zest, grated
1/4 cup olive oil
**Directions:**
In a salad bowl, combine the brown rice with the arugula, the beans and the

rest of the ingredients, toss and serve cold for breakfast.

**Nutrition:**
calories 473
fat 22fiber 7
carbs 53protein 13

## 32. Olive And Milk Bread
**Preparation time: 10 minutes**
**Cooking time: 50 minutes**
**Servings: 6**
**Ingredients:**
1 cup black olives, pitted, chopped
1 tablespoon olive oil
1/2 teaspoon fresh yeast
1/2 cup milk, preheated
1/2 teaspoon salt
1 teaspoon baking powder
2 cup wheat flour, whole grain
2 eggs, beaten
1 teaspoon butter, melted
1 teaspoon sugar
**Directions:**
In the big bowl combine together fresh yeast, sugar, and milk. Stir it until yeast is dissolved.
Then add salt, baking powder, butter, and eggs. Stir the dough mixture until homogenous and add 1 cup of wheat flour. Mix it up until smooth.
Add olives and remaining flour. Knead the non-sticky dough.
Transfer the dough into the non-sticky dough mold.
Bake the bread for 50 minutes at 350 F.

Check if the bread is cooked with the help of the toothpick. Is it is dry, the bread is cooked.
Remove the bread from the oven and let it chill for 10-15 minutes.
Remove it from the loaf mold and slice.

**Nutrition:**
calories 238

fat 7.7
fiber 1.9
carbs 35.5
protein 7.2

## 33. Breakfast Tostadas
**Preparation time: 10 minutes**
**Cooking time: 30 minutes**
**Servings: 6**
**Ingredients:**
1/2 white onion, diced
1 tomato, chopped
1 cucumber, chopped
1 tablespoon fresh cilantro, chopped
1/2 jalapeno pepper, chopped

1 tablespoon lime juice
6 corn tortillas
1 tablespoon canola oil
2 oz Cheddar cheese, shredded
1/2 cup white beans, canned, drained
6 eggs
1/2 teaspoon butter
1/2 teaspoon Sea salt
**Directions:**
Make Pico de Galo: in the salad bowl combine together diced white onion, tomato, cucumber, fresh cilantro, and jalapeno pepper.
Then add lime juice and a 1/2 tablespoon of canola oil. Mix up the mixture well. Pico de Galo is cooked.
After this, preheat the oven to 390F.
Line the tray with baking paper.
Arrange the corn tortillas on the baking paper and brush with remaining canola oil from both sides.
Bake the tortillas for 10 minutes or until they start to be crunchy.
Chill the cooked crunchy tortillas well.
Meanwhile, toss the butter in the skillet.

Crack the eggs in the melted butter and sprinkle them with sea salt.

Fry the eggs until the egg whites become white (cooked). Approximately for 3-5 minutes over the medium heat.

After this, mash the beans until you get puree texture.

Spread the bean puree on the corn tortillas.

Add fried eggs.

Then top the eggs with Pico de Galo and shredded Cheddar cheese.

**Nutrition:**

Calories 246

fat 11.1

fiber 4.7

carbs 24.5

protein 13.7

## 34. Chicken Souvlaki
**Preparation time:** 10 minutes
**Cooking time:** 2 minutes
**Servings:** 4
**Ingredients:**
4 pieces (6-inch) pitas, cut into halves
2 cups roasted chicken breast skinless, boneless, and sliced
1/4 cup red onion, thinly sliced
1/2 teaspoon dried oregano
1/2 cup Greek yogurt, plain
1/2 cup plum tomato, chopped
1/2 cup cucumber, peeled, chopped
1/2 cup (2 ounces) feta cheese, crumbled
1 tablespoon olive oil, extra-virgin, divided
1 tablespoon fresh dill, chopped
1 cup iceberg lettuce, shredded
1 1/4 teaspoons minced garlic, bottled, divided
**Directions:**
In a small mixing bowl, combine the yogurt, cheese, 1 teaspoon of the olive oil, and 1/4 teaspoon of the garlic until well mixed.
In a large skillet, heat the remaining olive oil over medium-high heat. Add the remaining 1 teaspoon garlic and the oregano; sauté for 20 seconds.
Add the chicken; cook for about 2 minutes or until the chicken are heated through.
Put 1/4 cup chicken into each pita halves. Top with 2 tablespoons yogurt mix, 2 tablespoons lettuce,1 tablespoon tomato, and 1 tablespoon cucumber. Divide the onion between the pita halves.
**Nutrition:**
Calories 414 fat 13.7 g
sodium 595 mg carb 38 g
fiber 2 g
protein.32.3 g

## 35. Tahini Pine Nuts Toast
**Preparation time:** 10 minutes
**Cooking time:** 0 minutes
**Servings:** 4
**Ingredients:**
2 whole wheat bread slices, toasted
1 teaspoon water
1 tablespoon tahini paste
2 teaspoons feta cheese, crumbled
Juice of 1/2 lemon
2 teaspoons pine nuts
A pinch of black pepper
**Directions:**
In a bowl, mix the tahini with the water and the lemon juice, whisk really well and spread over the toasted bread slices.
Top each serving with the remaining ingredients and serve for breakfast.
**Nutrition:**
calories 142
fat 7.6
fiber 2.7
carbs 13.7
protein 5.8

## 36. Eggs And Veggies
**Preparation time:** 10 minutes
**Cooking time:** 10 minutes
**Servings:** 4
**Ingredients:**
2 tomatoes, chopped
2 eggs, beaten - 1 bell pepper, chopped
1 teaspoon tomato paste
1/4 cup of water
1 teaspoon butter
1/2 white onion, diced
1/2 teaspoon chili flakes
1/3 teaspoon sea salt
**Directions:**
Put butter in the pan and melt it.
Add bell pepper and cook it for 3 minutes over the medium heat. Stir it from time to time.

After this, add diced onion and cook it for 2 minutes more.

Stir the vegetables and add tomatoes.

Cook them for 5 minutes over the medium-low heat.

Then add water and tomato paste. Stir well.

Add beaten eggs, chili flakes, and sea salt.

Stir well and cook menemen for 4 minutes over the medium-low heat.

The cooked meal should be half runny.

**Nutrition**:

calories 67fat 3.4

fiber 1.5carbs 6.4protein 3.8

### 37. Chili Scramble
**Preparation time: 10 minutes**
**Cooking time: 13 minutes**
**Servings: 4**
**Ingredients:**
3 tomatoes
4 eggs
1/4 teaspoon of sea salt
1/2 chili pepper, chopped
1 tablespoon butter
1 cup water, for cooking
**Directions:**
Pour water in the saucepan and bring it to boil.

Then remove water from the heat and add tomatoes.

Let the tomatoes stay in the hot water for 2-3 minutes.

After this, remove the tomatoes from water and peel them.

Place butter in the pan and melt it.

Add chopped chili pepper and fry it for 3 minutes over the medium heat.

Then chop the peeled tomatoes and add into the chili peppers.

Cook the vegetables for 5 minutes over the medium heat. Stir them from time to time.

After this, add sea salt and crack then eggs.

Stir (scramble) the eggs well with the help of the fork and cook them for 3 minutes over the medium heat.

**Nutrition**:
calories 105
fat 7.4
fiber 1.1
carbs 4
protein 6.4

### 38. Pear Oatmeal
**Preparation time: 10 minutes**
**Cooking time: 20 minutes**
**Servings: 4**
**Ingredients:**
1 cup oatmeal
1/3 cup milk
1 pear, chopped
1 teaspoon vanilla extract
1 tablespoon Splenda
1 teaspoon butter
1/2 teaspoon ground cinnamon
1 egg, beaten
**Directions:**
In the big bowl mix up together oatmeal, milk, egg, vanilla extract, Splenda, and ground cinnamon.

Melt butter and add it in the oatmeal mixture.

Then add chopped pear and stir it well.

Transfer the oatmeal mixture in the casserole mold and flatten gently.

Cover it with the foil and secure edges.

Bake the oatmeal for 25 minutes at 350F.

**Nutrition**:
calories 151
fat 3.9
fiber 3.3
carbs 23.6
protein 4.9

## 39. Olive Frittata

Preparation time: 10 minutes
Cooking time: 15 minutes
Servings: 5
Ingredients:
9 large eggs, lightly beaten
8 kalamata olives, pitted, chopped
1/4 cup olive oil
1/3 cup parmesan cheese, freshly grated
1/3 cup fresh basil, thinly sliced
1/2 teaspoon salt
1/2 teaspoon pepper
1/2 cup onion, chopped
1 sweet red pepper, diced
1 medium zucchini, cut to 1/2-inch cubes
1 package (4 ounce) feta cheese, crumbled

### Directions:

In a 10-inch oven-proof skillet, heat the olive oil until hot. Add the olives, zucchini, red pepper, and the onions, constantly stirring, until the vegetables are tender.

Ina bowl, mix the eggs, feta cheese, basil, salt, and pepper; pour in the skillet with vegetables. Adjust heat to medium-low, cover, and cook for about 10-12 minutes, or until the egg mixture is almost set.

Remove from the heat and sprinkle with the parmesan cheese. Transfer to the broiler.

With oven door partially open, broil 5 1/2 from the source of heat for about 2-3 minutes or until the top is golden. Cut into wedges.

Nutrition: :
Cal 288.5 total fat 22.8 g
carb 5.6 g fiber 1.2 g
sugar 3.3g
protein 15.2 g.

## 40. Mediterranean Egg Casserole

Preparation time: 10 minutes
Cooking time: 50 minutes
Servings: 4
Ingredients:
1 1/2 cups (6 ounces) feta cheese, crumbled
1 jar (6 ounces) marinated artichoke hearts, drained well, coarsely chopped
10 eggs
2 cups milk, low-fat
2 cups fresh baby spinach, packed, coarsely chopped
6 cups whole-wheat baguette, cut into 1-inch cubes
1 tablespoon garlic (about 4 cloves), finely chopped
1 tablespoon olive oil, extra-virgin
1/2 cup red bell pepper, chopped
1/2 cup Parmesan cheese, shredded
1/2 teaspoon pepper
1/2 teaspoon red pepper flakes
1/2 teaspoon salt
1/3 cup kalamata olives, pitted, halved
1/4 cup red onion, chopped
1/4 cup tomatoes (sun-dried) in oil, drained, chopped

### Directions:

Preheat oven to 350F.

Grease a 9x13-inch baking dish with olive oil cooking spray.

In an 8-inch non-stick pan over medium heat, heat the olive oil. Add the onions, garlic, and bell pepper; cook for about 3 minutes, frequently stirring, until slightly softened. Add the spinach; cook for about 1 minute or until starting to wilt.

Layer half of the baguette cubes in the preparation ared baking dish, then 1 cup of the eta, 1/4 cup Parmesan, the bell pepper mix, artichokes, the olives, and the tomatoes. Top with the remaining baguette cubes and then with the remaining 1/2 cup of feta.

In a large mixing bowl, whisk the eggs and the low-fat milk together. Beat in the pepper, salt and the pepper. Pour the mix over the bread layer in the baking dish, slightly pressing down. Sprinkle with the remaining 1/4 cup Parmesan.

Bake for about 40-45 minutes, or until the center is set and the top is golden brown. Before serving, let stand for 15 minutes.

**Nutrition:**
Cal 360
total fat 21 g
sodium 880 mg
carb 24 g
fiber 3 g
sugar 7 g
protein 20 g

## 41. Milk Scones

**Preparation time: 10 minutes**
**Cooking time: 10 minutes**
**Servings: 4**
**Ingredients:**
1/2 cup wheat flour, whole grain
1 teaspoon baking powder
1 tablespoon butter, melted
1 teaspoon vanilla extract
1 egg, beaten
3/4 teaspoon salt
3 tablespoons milk
1 teaspoon vanilla sugar
**Directions:**
In the mixing bowl combine together wheat flour, baking powder, butter, vanilla extract, and egg. Add salt and knead the soft and non-sticky dough. Add more flour if needed.
Then make the log from the dough and cut it into the triangles.
Line the tray with baking paper.

Arrange the dough triangles on the baking paper and transfer in the preheat to the 360F oven.
Cook the scones for 10 minutes or until they are light brown.
After this, chill the scones and brush with milk and sprinkle with vanilla sugar.
**Nutrition:**
calories 112fat 4.4
fiber 0.5
carbs 14.3
protein 3.4

## 42. Herbed Eggs And Mushroom Mix

**Preparation time: 10 minutes**
**Cooking time: 20 minutes**
**Servings: 4**
**Ingredients:**
1 red onion, chopped
1 bell pepper, chopped
1 tablespoon tomato paste
1/3 cup water
1/2 teaspoon of sea salt
1 tablespoon butter
1 cup cremini mushrooms, chopped
1 tablespoon fresh parsley
1 tablespoon fresh dill
1 teaspoon dried thyme
1/2 teaspoon dried oregano
1/2 teaspoon paprika
1/2 teaspoon chili flakes
1/2 teaspoon garlic powder
4 eggs
**Directions:**
Toss butter in the pan and melt it.
Then add chopped mushrooms and bell pepper. Roast the vegetables for 5 minutes over the medium heat. After this, add red onion and stir well.
Sprinkle the ingredients with garlic powder, chili flakes, dried oregano, and dried thyme. Mix up well
After this, add tomato paste and water.

Mix up the mixture until it is homogenous. Then add fresh parsley and dill. Cook the mixture for 5 minutes over the medium-high heat with the closed lid. After this, stir the mixture with the help of the spatula well.

Crack the eggs over the mixture and close the lid.

Cook shakshuka for 10 minutes over the low heat.

Nutrition: :calories 123, fat 7.5, fiber 1.7, carbs 7.8, protein 7.

## 43. Cherry Berry Bulgur Bowl
**Preparation Time: 15 minutes**
**Cooking Time: 15 minutes**
**Servings: 4**
**Ingredients:**
1 cup medium-grind bulgur
2 cups water - Pinch salt
1 cup halved and pitted cherries or 1 cup canned cherries, drained
1/2 cup raspberries
1/2 cup blackberries
1 tablespoon cherry jam
2 cups plain whole-milk yogurt
**Directions:**
Mix the bulgur, water, and salt in a medium saucepan. Do this in a medium heat. Bring to a boil.

Reduce the heat to low and simmer, partially covered, for 12 to 15 minutes or until the bulgur is almost tender. Cover, and let stand for 5 minutes to finish cooking do this after removing the pan from the heat.

While the bulgur is cooking, combine the raspberries and blackberries in a medium bowl. Stir the cherry jam into the fruit.

When the bulgur is tender, divide among four bowls. Top each bowl with 1/2 cup of yogurt and an equal amount of the berry mixture and serve.

**Nutrition:**
Calories: 242 Total fat: 6g
Saturated fat: 3g Sodium: 85mg
Phosphorus: 237mg Potassium: 438mg
Carbohydrates: 44g Fiber: 7g
Protein: 9g Sugar: 13g

## 44. Baked Curried Apple Oatmeal Cups
**Preparation Time: 10 minutes**
**Cooking Time: 20 minutes**
**Servings: 6**
**Ingredients:**
31/2 cups old-fashioned oats
3 tablespoons brown sugar
2 teaspoons of your preferred curry powder
1/8 teaspoon salt
1 cup unsweetened almond milk
1 cup unsweetened applesauce
1 teaspoon vanilla
1/2 cup chopped walnuts
**Directions:**
Preheat the oven to 375°F. Then spray a 12-cup muffin tin with baking spray then set aside.

Combine the oats, brown sugar, curry powder, and salt, and mix in a medium bowl.

Mix together the milk, applesauce, and vanilla in a small bowl,

Stir the liquid ingredients into the dry ingredients and mix until just combined. Stir in the walnuts.

Using a scant 1/3 cup for each divide the mixture among the muffin cups.

Bake this for 18 to 20 minutes until the oatmeal is firm. Serve.

**Nutrition:**
calories 243fat 20.2
fiber 1
carbs 2.8
protein 13.3

## 45. Pineapple, Macha & Beet Chia Pudding

**Preparation time: 10 minutes**
**Cooking time: 0 minutes**
**Servings: 4**
**Ingredients:**
1 cup chia seeds
1 teaspoon raw honey
2 cups almond milk
1 teaspoon matcha green tea powder
2 tablespoons fresh beetroot juice
1 whole pineapple
1 cup freshly squeezed lemon juice
1 knob of fresh ginger
Toasted almonds and figs to serve
**Directions:**
Green Chia pudding layer:
Add another half each of chia seeds, raw honey, almond milk, and matcha green tea powder to the blender and until very smooth, transfer to a bowl.
Beetroot layer: blend together beetroot and ginger with the remaining chia seeds, raw honey, vanilla, and coconut milk until very smooth; transfer to a separate bowl. In a food processor, puree the fresh pineapple until fine.
To assemble, layer the chia pudding in the bottom of serving glasses, followed by the pureed pineapple and then the beetroot layer. Top with figs and toasted almonds for a crunchy finish.

## 46. Coconut & Strawberry Smoothie Bowl

**Preparation time: 10 minutes**
**Cooking time: 0 minutes**
**Servings: 4**
**Ingredients:**
2 cups fresh strawberries
2 cups fresh spinach
1 cup coconut water
1 ripe banana
2 tablespoons raw pumpkin seeds

2 tablespoons chia seeds
1/2 cup coconut flakes, toasted
**Directions:**
In a blender, blend together almond milk, banana, and spinach until very smooth and creamy; add in strawberries and pulse to combine well.

Divide the smooth among serving bowls and top each serving with fresh strawberries, pumpkin seeds, chia seeds and toasted coconut flakes. Enjoy!

## 47. Farro Salad

**Preparation time: 10 minutes**
**Cooking time: 4 minutes**
**Servings: 2**
**Ingredients:**
1 tablespoon olive oil
A pinch of salt and black pepper
1 bunch baby spinach, chopped
1 avocado, pitted, peeled and chopped
1 garlic clove, minced
2 cups farro, already cooked
1/2 cup cherry tomatoes, cubed
**Directions:**
Heat up a pan with the oil over medium heat, add the spinach, and the rest of the ingredients, toss, cook for 4 minutes, divide into bowls and serve.
**Nutrition:** calories 157
fat 13.7
fiber 5.5
carbs 8.6
protein 3.6

## 48. Chili Avocado Scramble

**Preparation time: 10 minutes**
**Cooking time: 10 minutes**
**Servings: 4**
**Ingredients:**
4 eggs, beaten
1 white onion, diced
1 tablespoon avocado oil

1 avocado, finely chopped
1/2 teaspoon chili flakes
1 oz Cheddar cheese, shredded
1/2 teaspoon salt
1 tablespoon fresh parsley
**Directions:**
Pour avocado oil in the skillet and bring it to boil.
Then add diced onion and roast it until it is light brown.
Meanwhile, mix up together chili flakes, beaten eggs, and salt.
Pour the egg mixture over the cooked onion and cook the mixture for 1 minute over the medium heat.
After this, scramble the eggs well with the help of the fork or spatula. Cook the eggs until they are solid but soft.
After this, add chopped avocado and shredded cheese.
Stir the scramble well and transfer in the scrving plates.
Sprinkle the meal with fresh parsley.
**Nutrition:**
calories 236
fat 20.1
fiber 4
carbs 7.4
protein 8.6

## 49. Tapioca Pudding
**Preparation time: 10 minutes**
**Cooking time: 15 minutes**
**Servings: 3**
**Ingredients:**
1/4 cup pearl tapioca
1/4 cup maple syrup
2 cups almond milk
1/2 cup coconut flesh, shredded
1 and 1/2 teaspoon lemon juice
**Directions:**
In a pan, combine the milk with the tapioca and the rest of the ingredients, bring to a simmer over medium heat, and cook for 15 minutes.

Divide the mix into bowls, cool it down and serve for breakfast.
**Nutrition:**
calories 361
fat 28.5
fiber 2.7
carbs 28.3
protein 2.8

## 50. Feta And Eggs Mix
**Preparation time: 10 minutes**
**Cooking time: 5 minutes**
**Servings: 4**
**Ingredients:**
4 eggs, beaten
1/2 teaspoon ground black pepper
2 oz Feta, scrambled
1/2 teaspoon salt
1 teaspoon butter
1 teaspoon fresh parsley, chopped
**Directions:**
Melt butter in the skillet and add beaten eggs.
Then add parsley, salt, and scrambled eggs. Cook the eggs for 1 minute over the high heat.
Add ground black pepper and scramble eggs with the help of the fork.

Cook the eggs for 3 minutes over the medium-high heat.
**Nutrition:**
calories 110
fat 8.4
fiber 0.1
carbs 1.1
protein 7.6

## 51. Banana pancakes
**Preparation time: 10 minutes**
**Cooking time: 20 minutes**
**Servings: 4**
**Ingredients**
1 cup whole wheat flour
1/4 tsp baking soda

1/4 tsp baking powder
1 cup mashed banana
2 eggs
1 cup milk

**Directions**

In a bowl combine all ingredients together and mix well

In a skillet heat olive oil

Pour 1/4 of the batter and cook each pancake for 1-2 minutes per side

When ready remove from heat and serve

**Nutrition:**

carbs 7g
 fat 14g
protein 15g
Calories 210

## 52. Nectarine pancakes

**Preparation time: 10 minutes**
**Cooking time: 30 minutes**
**Servings: 4**
**Ingredients**
1 cup whole wheat flour
1/4 tsp baking soda
1/4 tsp baking powder
1 cup nectarines
2 eggs
1 cup milk

**Directions**

In a bowl combine all ingredients together and mix well

In a skillet heat olive oil

Pour 1/4 of the batter and cook each pancake for 1-2 minutes per side

When ready remove from heat and serve

**Nutrition:**

carbs 7g fat 14g
protein 15g
Calories 210

## 53. Pancakes

**Preparation time: 10 minutes**
**Cooking time: 30 minutes**

**Servings: 4**
**Ingredients:**
1 cup whole wheat flour
1/4 tsp baking soda
1/4 tsp baking powder
2 eggs
1 cup milk

**Directions:**

In a bowl combine all ingredients together and mix well

In a skillet heat olive oil

Pour 1/4 of the batter and cook each pancake for 1-2 minutes per side

When ready remove from heat and serve

**Nutrition:**

carbs 2g
 fat 6g
protein 10g
Calories 100 g

## 54. Peaches muffins

**Preparation time: 10 minutes**
**Cooking time: 30 minutes**
**Servings: 4**
**Ingredients**
2 eggs
1 tablespoon olive oil
1 cup milk
2 cups whole wheat flour
1 tsp baking soda
1/4 tsp baking soda
1 cup peaches
1 tsp cinnamon
1/4 cup molasses

**Directions**

In a bowl combine all wet ingredients

In another bowl combine all dry ingredients

Combine wet and dry ingredients together

Pour mixture into 8-12 preparation ared muffin cups, fill 2/3 of the cups

Bake for 18-20 minutes at 375 F, when ready remove and serve
**Nutrition:**
carbs 2g
fat 6g
protein 10g
Calories 100

## 55. Lemon muffins
**Preparation time: 10 minutes**
**Cooking time: 30 minutes**
**Servings: 4**
**Ingredients**
2 eggs
1 tablespoon olive oil
1 cup milk
2 cups whole wheat flour
1 tsp baking soda
1/4 tsp baking soda
1 tsp cinnamon
1 cup lemon slices
**Directions**
In a bowl combine all wet ingredients
In another bowl combine all dry ingredients
Combine wet and dry ingredients together
Pour mixture into 8-12 preparation ared muffin cups, fill 2/3 of the cups
Bake for 18-20 minutes at 375 F
When ready remove from the oven and serve
**Nutrition:**
carbs 2g
fat 6g
 protein 10g
Calories 100

## 56. Blueberry muffins
**Preparation time: 10 minutes**
**Cooking time: 30 minutes**
**Servings: 4**
**Ingredients**
2 eggs
1 tablespoon olive oil

1 cup milk
2 cups whole wheat flour
1 tsp baking soda
1/4 tsp baking soda
1 tsp cinnamon
1 cup blueberries
**Directions**
In a bowl combine all wet ingredients
In another bowl combine all dry ingredients
Combine wet and dry ingredients together
Fold in blueberries and mix well
Pour mixture into 8-12 preparation ared muffin cups, fill 2/3 of the cups
Bake for 18-20 minutes at 375 F, when ready remove and serve
**Nutrition:**
carbs 2g
fat 6g
protein 10g
Calories 100

## 57. Kumquat muffins
**Preparation time: 10 minutes**
**Cooking time: 30 minutes**
**Servings: 4**
**Ingredients**
2 eggs
1 tablespoon olive oil
1 cup milk
2 cups whole wheat flour
1 tsp baking soda
1/4 tsp baking soda
1 tsp cinnamon
1 cup kumquat
**Directions**
In a bowl combine all wet ingredients
In another bowl combine all dry ingredients
Combine wet and dry ingredients together
Pour mixture into 8-12 preparation ared muffin cups, fill 2/3 of the cups
Bake for 18-20 minutes at 375 F

When ready remove from the oven and serve

**Nutrition:**

carbs 2g

fat 6g

protein 10g

Calories 100

## 58. Chocolate muffins

**Preparation time: 10 minutes**

**Cooking time: 30 minutes**

**Servings: 7**

**Ingredients**

2 eggs

1 tablespoon olive oil

1 cup milk

2 cups whole wheat flour

1 tsp baking soda

1/4 tsp baking soda

1 tsp cinnamon

1 cup chocolate chips

**Directions**

In a bowl combine all dry ingredients

In another bowl combine all dry ingredients

Combine wet and dry ingredients together

Fold in chocolate chips and mix well

Pour mixture into 8-12 preparation ared muffin cups, fill 2/3 of the cups

Bake for 18-20 minutes at 375 F, when ready remove and serve

**Nutrition:**

carbs 2g

fat 6g

protein 10g

Calories 100

## 59. Muffins

**Preparation time: 10 minutes**

**Cooking time: 20 minutes**

**Servings: 4**

**Ingredients**

2 eggs

1 tablespoon olive oil

1 cup milk

2 cups whole wheat flour

1 tsp baking soda

1/4 tsp baking soda

1 tsp cinnamon

**Directions**

In a bowl combine all wet ingredients

In another bowl combine all dry ingredients

Combine wet and dry ingredients together

Pour mixture into 8-12 preparation ared muffin cups, fill 2/3 of the cups

Bake for 18-20 minutes at 375 F

When ready remove from the oven and serve

**Nutrition:**

carbs 2g

 fat 6g

protein 10g

Calories 100

## 60. Omelette

**Preparation time: 10 minutes**

**Cooking time: 15 minutes**

**Servings: 4**

**Ingredients**

2 eggs

1/4 tsp salt

1/4 tsp black pepper

1 tablespoon olive oil

1/4 cup cheese

1/4 tsp basil

**Directions**

In a bowl combine all ingredients together and mix well

In a skillet heat olive oil and pour the egg mixture

Cook for 1-2 minutes per side

When ready remove omelette from the skillet and serve

**Nutrition:**

carbs 2g fat 6g

protein 10g

Calories 100

## 61. Onion Omelette

**Preparation Time: 15 Minutes**
**Cooking Time:** 25 Minutes
**Servings: 3**
**Ingredients:**
2 eggs
1/4 tsp salt
1/4 tsp black pepper
1 tablespoon olive oil
1/4 cup cheese
1/4 tsp basil
1 cup red onion

**Directions:**
In a bowl combine all ingredients together and mix well
In a skillet heat olive oil and pour the egg mixture
Cook for 1-2 minutes per side
When ready remove omelette from the skillet and serve

**Nutrition:**
carbs 50g
fat 11g
protein 10g
Calories 320

## 62. Broccoli Omelette

**Preparation Time: 15 Minutes**
**Cooking Time:** 25 Minutes
**Servings: 3**
**Ingredients:**
2 eggs
1/4 tsp salt
1/4 tsp black pepper
1 tablespoon olive oil
1/4 cup cheese
1/4 tsp basil
1 cup broccoli
**Directions:**
In a bowl combine all ingredients together and mix well
In a skillet heat olive oil and pour the egg mixture

Cook for 1-2 minutes per side
When ready remove omelette from the skillet and serve
**Nutrition:**
carbs 50g
fat 11g
protein 10g
Calories 320

## 63. Beets Omelette

**Preparation Time: 15 Minutes**
**Cooking Time:** 25 Minutes
**Servings: 3**
**Ingredients:**
2 eggs
1/4 tsp salt
1/4 tsp black pepper
1 tablespoon olive oil
1/4 cup cheese
1/4 tsp basil
1 cup beets
**Directions:**
In a bowl combine all ingredients together and mix well
In a skillet heat olive oil and pour the egg mixture
Cook for 1-2 minutes per side
When ready remove omelette from the skillet and serve
**Nutrition:**
carbs 50g
fat 11g
protein 10g
Calories 320

## 64. Breakfast Beans

**Preparation Time: 15 Minutes**
**Cooking Time:** 25 Minutes
**Servings: 3**
**Ingredients:**
1 (15-oz.) can chickpeas, rinsed and drained
1 (15-oz.) can fava beans, rinsed and drained
1 cup water

1 TB. minced garlic
1 tsp. salt
1/2 cup fresh lemon juice
1/2 tsp. cayenne
1/2 cup fresh parsley, chopped
1 large tomato, diced
3 medium radishes, sliced
1/4 cup extra-virgin olive oil

**Directions:**

In a 2-quart pot over medium-low heat, combine chickpeas, fava beans, and water. Simmer for 10 minutes.

Pour bean mixture into a large bowl, and add garlic, salt, and lemon juice. Stir and smash half of beans with the back of a wooden spoon.

Sprinkle cayenne over beans, and evenly distribute parsley, tomatoes, and radishes over top. Drizzle with extra-virgin olive oil and serve warm or at room temperature.

**Nutrition:**

carbs 35g
fat 30g
protein 20g
Calories 460

## 65. Seeds and Lentils Oats

**Preparation Time: 15 Minutes**
**Cooking Time:** 25 Minutes
**Servings: 3**
**Ingredients:**

1/2 cup red lentils
1/4 cup pumpkin seeds, toasted
2 teaspoons olive oil
1/4 cup rolled oats
1/4 cup coconut flesh, shredded
1 tablespoon honey
1 tablespoon orange zest, grated
1 cup Greek yogurt
1 cup blackberries

**Directions:**

Spread the lentils on a baking sheet lined with parchment paper, introduce

in the oven and roast at 370 degrees F for 30 minutes.

Add the rest of the ingredients except the yogurt and the berries, toss and bake at 370 degrees F for 20 minutes more.

Transfer this to a bowl, add the rest of the ingredients, toss, divide into smaller bowls and serve for breakfast.

**Nutrition:**

calories 204
fat 7.1
fiber 10.4
carbs 27.6
protein 9.5

## 66. Couscous with Artichokes, Sun-dried Tomatoes and Feta

**Preparation Time: 15 Minutes**
**Cooking Time:** 25 Minutes
**Servings: 3**
**Ingredients:**

3 cups chicken breast, cooked, chopped
2 1/3 cups water, divided
2 jars (6-ounces each) marinated artichoke hearts, undrained
1/4 teaspoon black pepper, freshly ground
1/2 cup tomatoes, sun-dried
1/2 cup (2 ounces) feta cheese, crumbled
1 cup flat-leaf parsley, fresh, chopped
1 3/4 cups whole-wheat Israeli couscous, uncooked
1 can (14 1/2 ounces) vegetable broth

**Directions:**

In a microwavable bowl, combine 2 cups of the water and the tomatoes. Microwave on HIGH for about 3 minutes or until the water boils. When water is boiling, remove from the microwave, cover, and let stand for about 3 minutes or until the tomatoes are soft; drain, chop, and set aside.

In a large saucepan, place the vegetable broth and the remaining 1/3 cup of water; bring to boil. Stir in the couscous, cover, reduce heat, and simmer for about 8 minutes or until tender. Remove the pan from the heat; add the tomatoes and the remaining ingredients. Stir to combine.

**Nutrition:**
Cal 419
total fat 14.1 g
chol 64 mg.
sodium 677 mg
carb 42.5 g
fiber 2.6 g
protein 30.2 g.

# CHAPTER 11:

# Shake And Smoothie Recipes

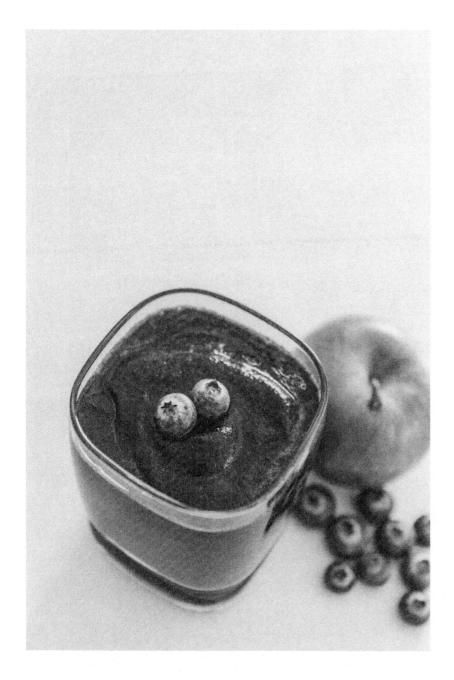

## 67. Ginger Citrus Liver Detox Drink

**Preparation Time:** 10 minutes
**Cooking Time:** 0 minutes
**Servings:** 1
**Ingredients**
1 lemon, peeled
1-inch knob fresh ginger root, finely grated
1 orange, peeled
1 grapefruit, peeled
A pinch of cayenne pepper
**Directions**
Juice all the ingredients in a juicer, except cayenne pepper; stir in cayenne pepper and serve.
**Nutrition:**
Calories: 11;  Total Fat: 0 g;  Carbs: 0 g;
Dietary Fiber: 0 g;
Sugars: 1 g;  Protein: 5 g;
Cholesterol: 0 mg;  Sodium: 2 mg

## 68. Ginger, Pineapple & Kale Detox Juice

**Preparation Time:** 10 minutes
**Cooking Time:** 0 minutes
**Servings:** 1
**Ingredients**
1/4 medium pineapple
1 lemon, peeled
1-inch fresh ginger
2 large cucumbers
1 cup chopped kale
1/2 cup fresh mint
**Directions**
Juice all the ingredients, one at a time, in a juicer and serve.
**Nutrition:**
Calories: 125;  Total Fat: 0.8 g;
Carbs: 30.2 g;  Dietary Fiber: 7.4 g;
Sugars: 10.5 g;
Protein: 5.1 g;
Cholesterol: 0 mg;

Sodium: 46 mg

## 69. Beet Citrus Cleanser

**Preparation Time:** 10 minutes
**Cooking Time:** 0 minutes
**Servings:** 2
**Ingredients**
2 beets
1 tangerine
1 orange
1 lime
2 carrots
2 cups dandelion greens
2-inch knob ginger
**Directions**
Add all ingredients to the juicer and juice. Enjoy!
**Nutrition:**
Calories: 173;
Total Fat: 0.9 g;  Carbs: 41.6 g;
Dietary Fiber: 9.4 g;  Sugars: 25.1 g;
Protein: 5.2 g;  Cholesterol: 0 mg;
Sodium: 163 mg

## 70. Super Detox Green Juice

**Preparation Time:** 10 minutes
**Cooking Time:** 0 minutes
**Servings:** 1
**Ingredients**
1 apple, seeded, cored, chopped
1 lemon peeled
1 cup spinach
2 kale leaves
1 cucumber, chopped
2 celery stalks, chopped
Handful of fresh parsley or cilantro
2 teaspoons chia seeds
**Directions**
Add all ingredients, except chia seed, to the juicer and juice; stir in the chia seeds and drink.
**Nutrition:**
Calories: 158;  Total Fat: 1 g;
Carbs: 39 g;  Dietary Fiber: 9 g;
Sugars: 20 g;  Protein: 5 g;

Cholesterol: 0 mg;
Sodium: 112 mg

## 71. Refreshing Carrot Detoxifier

**Preparation Time: 10 minutes**
**Cooking Time: 0 minutes**
**Servings: 2**
**Ingredients**
4 carrots
1 cup sprouts
1-cm fresh ginger
1 kiwi fruit
1 lemon
1 green apple
1 cucumber
2 stalks celery
1 cup parsley
**Directions**
Add all ingredients to the juicer and juice. Enjoy!
**Nutrition:**
Calories: 173;
Total Fat: 0.8 g;
Carbs: 42.3 g;
Dietary Fiber: 9.5 g;
Sugars: 23.8 g;
Protein: 1.4 g;
Cholesterol: 0 mg;
Sodium: 126 mg

## 72. Super Cleanser Juice

**Preparation Time: 10 minutes**
**Cooking Time: 0 minutes**
**Servings: 1**
**Ingredients**
1/4 cup fresh aloe vera juice
1 lemon, peeled
5 asparagus spears
1 cucumber
10 stalks celery
Handful of cilantro
Handful of parsley
**Directions**

Add all ingredients to the juicer and juice. Enjoy!

**Nutrition:**
Calories: 113;
Total Fat: 0.9 g;
Carbs: 26.1 g;
Dietary Fiber: 8.4 g;
Sugars: 11 g;
Protein: 6.4 g;
Cholesterol: 0 mg;
Sodium: 160 mg

## 73. Ginger, Pineapple & Cabbage Detoxifier

**Preparation Time: 10 minutes**
**Cooking Time: 0 minutes**
**Servings: 1**
**Ingredients**
1/4 medium pineapple
1 lemon, peeled
1-inch fresh ginger
2 large cucumbers
1 cup chopped cabbage
1/2 cup fresh mint
**Directions**
Juice all the ingredients, one at a time, in a juicer and serve.
**Nutrition:**
Calories: 125;
Total Fat: 0.8 g;
Carbs: 30.2 g;
Dietary Fiber: 7.4 g;
Sugars: 10.5 g;
Protein: 5.1 g;
Cholesterol: 0 mg;
Sodium: 46 mg

## 74. Ultimate Toxin Flush Shot

**Preparation Time: 15 Minutes**
**Cooking Time: 0 minutes**
**Servings: 1**
**Ingredients**

1 knob of ginger
1 cup water
2 tablespoons fresh lemon juice
1/2 teaspoon cayenne pepper
1 teaspoon turmeric
1/2 teaspoon pepper
1 teaspoon raw honey
ice

**Directions**

Juice ginger through a juicer; stir in water, fresh lemon juice, cayenne, turmeric, black pepper, raw honey, and ice. Enjoy!

**Nutrition:**
Calories: 153
Total Fat: 6 g
Carbs: 17 g
Dietary Fiber: 1 g
Sugars: 2 g
Protein: 8 g
Cholesterol: 0 mg
Sodium: 12 mg

## 75. Detoxifying Vegetable Juice

**Preparation Time: 10 minutes**
**Cooking Time: 0 minutes**
**Servings: 1**
**Ingredients**
1/2 cup chopped kale
1/2 cup baby spinach
1 cucumber
1-inch ginger
2 carrots
1 pear
1/2 apple
2 celery stalks

**Directions**

Add all ingredients to the juicer and juice. Enjoy!

**Nutrition:**
Calories: 259;
Total Fat: 0.8 g;
Carbs: 64.6 g;
Dietary Fiber: 12.9 g;

Sugars: 36.7 g;
Protein: 5.4 g;
Cholesterol: 0 mg;
Sodium: 160 mg

## 76. Hot Golden Elixir

**Preparation Time: 15 Minutes**
**Cooking Time: 0 minutes**
**Servings: 1**
**Ingredients**
1/4 cup fresh lemon juice
1 cup hot water
1 teaspoon raw honey
1/4 teaspoon cayenne pepper
1/8 teaspoon ground ginger
1/8 teaspoon turmeric

**Directions**

In a mug, stir everything together until well blended. Enjoy!

**Nutrition:**
Calories: 39;  Total Fat: 0.6 g;
Carbs: 7.6 g;  Dietary Fiber: 0.5 g;
Sugars: 7.1 g;  Protein: 0.6 g;
Cholesterol: 0 mg;
Sodium: 20 mg

## 77. Ultimate Liver Detox Juice

**Preparation Time: 15 minutes**
**Cooking Time: 0 minutes**
**Servings: 1**
**Ingredients:**
3 carrots, peeled
1 beet, peeled
2 red apples, chopped
1/2 lemon, peeled
1/2 inch ginger root
6 kale leaves
1 cup chopped cabbage

**Directions:**

Place all the ingredients in a juicer and juice. Stir to mix well and serve with ice cubes.

**Nutrition:**
Calories: 232;  Total Fat: 0.6 g;

Carbs: 57.4 g;
Dietary Fiber:11.2 g;
Sugars: 33.2 g;
Protein: 5.4 g; Cholesterol: 0 mg;
Sodium: 147 mg

## 78. Raspberry Peach Breakfast Smoothie

**Preparation Time: 15 Minutes**
**Cooking Time: 1 minute**
**Servings: 2**
**Ingredients:**
1/3 cup of raspberries, (it can be frozen)
1/2 peach, skin and pit removed
1 tablespoon of honey
1 cup of coconut water
**Directions:**
Mix all ingredients together and blend it until smooth.
Pour and serve chilled in a tall glass or mason jar.
**Nutrition:**
Calories: 86.3 kcal
Carbohydrate: 20.6 g
Protein: 1.4 g
Sodium: 3 mg
Potassium: 109 mg
Phosphorus: 36.08 mg
Dietary Fiber: 2.6 g
Fat: 0.31 g

## 79. Charcoal Black Lemonade

**Preparation Time: 10 minutes**
**Cooking Time: 0 minutes**
**Servings: 4**
**Ingredients**
1 capsule activated charcoal
1/4 cup fresh lemon juice
4 cups filtered water
2 tablespoons raw honey
**Directions**

In a large bowl, whisk all the ingredients together until well blended. Serve over ice.
**Nutrition:**
Calories: 117; Total Fat: 0.5 g;
Carbs: 11.5 g; Dietary Fiber: 0 g;
Sugars: 7.3 g; Protein: 0.5 g;
Cholesterol: 32 mg;
Sodium: 73 mg

## 80. Cantaloupe Blackberry Smoothie

**Preparation Time: 15 Minutes**
**Cooking Time: 5 minutes**
**Servings: 2**
**Ingredients:**
1 cup coconut milk yogurt
1/2 cup blackberries
2 cups fresh cantaloupe
1 banana
**Directions:**
Toss all your ingredients into your blender then process till smooth.
Serve and enjoy.
**Nutrition:**
Calories: 160
Fat: 4.5g
Carbs: 33.7g
Protein: 1.8g
Fiber: 0g

## 81. Cantaloupe Kale Smoothie

**Preparation Time: 15 Minutes**
**Cooking Time: 5 minutes**
**Servings: 2**
**Ingredients:**
8 oz. water
1 orange, peeled
3 cups kale, chopped
1 banana, peeled
2 cups cantaloupe, chopped
1 zucchini, chopped
**Directions:**

Toss all your ingredients into your blender then process till smooth and creamy.

Serve immediately and enjoy.

**Nutrition:**
Calories: 203
Fat: 0.5g.
Carbs: 49.2g.
Protein: 5.6g.
Fiber: 0g.

## 82. Mix Berry Cantaloupe Smoothie

**Preparation Time: 15 Minutes**
**Cooking Time: 5 minutes**
**Servings: 2**
**Ingredients:**
1 cup alkaline water
2 fresh Seville orange juices
1/4 cup fresh mint leaves
1 1/2 cups mixed berries
2 cups cantaloupe
**Directions:**
Toss all your ingredients into your blender then process till smooth.
Serve immediately and enjoy.
**Nutrition:**
Calories: 122
Fat: 1g.
Carbs: 26.1g.
Protein: 2.4g.
Fiber: 0g.

## 83. Avocado Kale Smoothie

**Preparation Time: 15 Minutes.**
**Cooking Time: 5 minutes.**
**Servings: 3**
**Ingredients:**
1 cup water
1/2 Seville orange, peeled
1 avocado
1 cucumber, peeled
1 cup kale
1 cup ice cubes
**Directions:**

Toss all your ingredients into your blender then process till smooth and creamy.

Serve immediately and enjoy.

**Nutrition:**
Calories: 160
Fat: 13.3g.
Carbs: 11.6g.
Protein: 2.4g.
Fiber: 0g.

## 84. Apple Kale Cucumber Smoothie

**Preparation Time: 15 Minutes.**
**Cooking Time: 5 minutes.**
**Servings: 1**
**Ingredients:**
3/4 cup water
1/2 green apple, diced
3/4 cup kale
1/2 cucumber
**Directions:**
Toss all your ingredients into your blender then process till smooth and creamy.
Serve immediately and enjoy.
**Nutrition:**
Calories: 86
Fat: 0.5g.
Carbs: 21.7g.
Protein: 1.9g.
Fiber: 0g.

## 85. Refreshing Cucumber Smoothie

**Preparation Time: 15 Minutes.**
**Cooking Time: 5 minutes.**
**Servings: 2**
**Ingredients:**
1 cup ice cubes
20 drops liquid stevia
2 fresh lime, peeled and halved
1 tsp. lime zest, grated
1 cucumber, chopped
1 avocado, pitted and peeled

2 cups kale
1 tbsp. creamed coconut
3/4 cup coconut water

**Directions:**

Toss all your ingredients into your blender then process till smooth and creamy.

Serve immediately and enjoy.
**Nutrition:**
Calories: 313
Fat: 25.1g.
Carbs: 24.7g.
Protein: 4.9g.
Fiber: 0g.

## 86. Cauliflower Veggie Smoothie
**Preparation Time: 15 Minutes**
**Cooking Time: 5 minutes**
**Servings: 4**
**Ingredients:**
1 zucchini, peeled and chopped
1 Seville orange, peeled
1 apple, diced
1 banana
1 cup kale
1/2 cup cauliflower
**Directions:**
Toss all your ingredients into your blender then process till smooth and creamy.
Serve immediately and enjoy.
**Nutrition:**
Calories: 71
Fat: 0.3g.
Carbs: 18.3g.
Protein: 1.3g.
Fiber: 0g.

## 87. Soursop Smoothie
**Preparation Time: 15 Minutes**
**Cooking Time: 5 minutes**
**Servings: 2**
**Ingredients:**
3 quartered frozen Burro Bananas
1-1/2 cups of Homemade Coconut Milk
1/4 cup of Walnuts
1 teaspoon of Sea Moss Gel
1 teaspoon of Ground Ginger
1 teaspoon of Soursop Leaf Powder
1 handful of Kale
**Directions:**
Prepare and put all ingredients in a blender or a food processor.
Blend it well until you reach a smooth consistency.
Serve and enjoy your Soursop Smoothie!
Useful Tips:
If you don't have frozen Bananas, you can use fresh ones.
**Nutrition:**
Calories: 213
Fat: 3.1g.
Carbs: 6g.
Protein: 8g.
Fiber: 4.3g.

## 88. Magical Liver Elixir
**Preparation Time: 10 minutes**
**Cooking Time: 0 minutes**
**Servings: 1**
**Ingredients**
2 knobs of fresh turmeric
2-inch piece of fresh ginger root
2 garlic cloves
2 red onions
1 cup spinach
4 celery stalks
1 carrot
**Directions**
Wash and run all ingredients through a juicer. Serve right away.
**Nutrition:**
Calories: 164;
Total Fat: 1.2 g;
Carbs: 36.2 g;
Dietary Fiber: 9 g;
Sugars: 13.7 g;
Protein: 4.4 g;
Cholesterol: 0 mg;
Sodium: 109 mg

## 89. Chilled Toxin Flush Detox Drink

**Preparation Time: 15 minutes**
**Cooking Time: 15 minutes**
**Servings: 6**
**Ingredients**
6 tea bags
1/2 cup fresh mint leaves
3 lemons, sliced
3 limes, sliced
3 oranges, sliced
6 cups water
1 teaspoon liquid stevia
1 handful ice cubes
**Directions**
Mix lemon slices, lime slices, orange slices, mint leaves and water in a large teapot; bring to a rolling boil and simmer for about 10 minutes; let cool and strain the mixture through a fine mesh and stir in stevia. Serve over ice.
**Nutrition:**
Calories: 24;
Total Fat: 0 g;
Carbs: 4.2 g;
Dietary Fiber: 0.5 g;
Sugars: 1.6 g;
Protein: 0 g;
Cholesterol: 0 mg;
Sodium: 7 mg

## 90. Liver Detox Juice

**Preparation Time: 10 minutes**
**Cooking Time: 0 minutes**
**Servings: 1**
**Ingredients**
1 orange, peeled
1 cucumber
1 cup watercress leaves
2 garlic cloves
6 leaves kale
5 stalks celery
1-inch fresh ginger
Dash of cayenne

**Directions**
Add all ingredients to the juicer and juice. Enjoy!
**Nutrition:**
Calories: 206;
Total Fat: 0.3 g;
Carbs: 47.4 g;
Dietary Fiber: 11.2 g;
Sugars: 25.9 g;
Protein: 9.3 g;
Cholesterol: 0 mg;
Sodium: 160 mg

## 91. Ginger Radish Zinger

**Preparation Time: 10 minutes**
**Cooking Time: 0 minutes**
**Servings: 1**
**Ingredients**
1 lemon
1/2 green apple
1 cups spinach
1 radish
2 stalks celery
1.5-cm ginger
1/2 cup parsley
**Directions**
Add all ingredients to the juicer and juice. Enjoy!
**Nutrition:**
Calories: 150;
Total Fat: 0.2 g;
Carbs: 36.7 g;
Dietary Fiber: 8.7 g;
Sugars: 9.1 g;
Protein: 5.7 g;
Cholesterol: 0 mg;
Sodium: 100 mg

## 92. Ginger Pineapple Drink

**Preparation Time: 15 Minutes**
**Cooking Time: 0 minutes**
**Servings: 2**
**Ingredients**
1-inch piece fresh ginger

1/2 cup pineapple chunks
2 tablespoons lime juice
1 apple, diced
1/2 cup mango chunks

**Directions**

Blend together all ingredients until smooth. Serve over ice.

**Nutrition:**

Calories: 186;
Total Fat: 0.8 g;
Carbs: 47.2 g;
Dietary Fiber: 6.6 g;
Protein: 1.8 g;
Cholesterol: 0 mg;
Sodium: 6 mg;
Sugars: 28.7 g

## 93. Detoxifying Turmeric Tea

**Preparation Time: 10 minutes**
**Cooking Time: 0 minutes**
**Servings: 1**
**Ingredients**

1 1/2 cups boiling water
1 bag of chamomile tea
1 bag of peppermint tea
1/2 teaspoon vanilla extract
1 teaspoon turmeric
1 teaspoon ginger
1/4 teaspoon pepper
1 teaspoon raw honey

**Directions**

In a large mug, combine hot water, chamomile and peppermint teas and let steep for at least 3 minutes; stir in the remaining ingredients and serve hot!

**Nutrition:**

Calories: 116;
Total Fat: 7 g;
Carbs: 13 g;
Dietary Fiber: 1 g;
Sugars: 2 g
Protein: 17 g;
Cholesterol: 0 mg;
Sodium: 13 mg

## 94. Lemon Ginger Detox Juice

**Preparation Time: 10 minutes**
**Cooking Time: 0 minutes**
**Servings: 1**
**Ingredients**

1 lemon, peeled
1-inch knob fresh ginger root, finely grated
1 orange, peeled
1 grapefruit, peeled
1 garlic clove
A pinch of cayenne pepper

**Directions**

Juice all the ingredients in a juicer, except cayenne pepper; stir in cayenne pepper and serve.

**Nutrition:**

Calories: 11;
Total Fat: 0 g;
Carbs: 0 g;
Dietary Fiber: 0 g;
Sugars: 1 g;
Protein: 5 g;
Cholesterol: 0 mg;
Sodium: 2 mg

## 95. Ginger Pineapple Detox Drink

**Preparation Time: 10 minutes**
**Cooking Time: 0 minutes**
**Servings: 1**
**Ingredients**

1 pineapple center
1-inch ginger root
2 carrots
3 celery stalks
Handful mint leaves
Small handful of cilantro

**Directions**
Juice all the ingredients in a juicer and serve.
**Nutrition:**
Calories: 152;
Total Fat: 0.5 g;
Carbs: 37.2 g;
Dietary Fiber: 6.8 g;
Sugars: 23.3 g;
Protein: 2.8 g;
Cholesterol: 0 mg;
Sodium: 137 mg

## 96. Chilled Ginger Citrus Drink
**Preparation Time: 10 minutes**
**Cooking Time: 0 minutes**
**Servings: 1**
**Ingredients**
1 knob fresh ginger
1 large grapefruit
1 orange
1 lemon
**Directions**
Juice ginger and red grapefruit and orange; set aside. Squeeze in the lemon juice and stir to combine well. Refrigerate until chilled before serving.
**Nutrition:**
Calories: 193;
Total Fat: 0.6 g;
Carbs: 48.6g;
Dietary Fiber: 8.1g;
Protein: 3.8g;
Cholesterol: 0mg;
Sodium: 0mg;
Sugars: 40.4g

## 97. Avocado Smoothie
**Preparation Time: 10 minutes**
**Cooking Time: 0 minutes**
**Servings: 1**
**Ingredients**
1 Banana

2 tablespoons cacao powder
 tsp coconut oil
1 avocado
1 tsp vanilla extract
2 tablespoons honey
1 cup ice

**Directions**
In a blender place all ingredients and blend until smooth
Pour smoothie in a glass and serve
**Nutrition:**
324 Calories
24g fat
20g protein
7g carbs

## 98. Breakfast Smoothie
**Preparation Time: 10 minutes**
**Cooking Time: 0 minutes**
**Servings: 1**
**Ingredients**
**1 banana**
1 tsp coffee
1 tsp cinnamon
1 tsp honey
**1 cup milk**
**Directions**
In a blender place all ingredients and blend until smooth
Pour smoothie in a glass and serve
**Nutrition:**
calories 144
fat 7.7
fiber 1.4
carbs 6.3 protein 5.5

## 99. Banana Smoothie
**Preparation Time: 10 minutes**
**Cooking Time: 0 minutes**
**Servings: 1**
**Ingredients**
2 tablespoons cocoa powder
**1 cup ice**
**1 banana**

1 cup skimmed milk
**Directions**
In a blender place all ingredients and blend until smooth
Pour smoothie in a glass and serve
**Nutrition:**
calories 221
fat 12.2
fiber 0.1
carbs 5.4
protein 1

## 100. Green Smoothie
**Preparation Time: 10 minutes**
**Cooking Time: 0 minutes**
**Servings: 1**
**Ingredients**
**1 banana**
**1 apple**
**1 kiwi**
2 oz. spinach

**Directions**
In a blender place all ingredients and blend until smooth
Pour smoothie in a glass and serve

**Nutrition:**
Calories 128
Fat 9.4 g
Carbohydrates 10.4 g
Sugar 4 g

## 101. Kale Smoothie
**Preparation Time: 10 minutes**
**Cooking Time: 0 minutes**
**Servings: 1**
**Ingredients**
2 oz. spinach leaves
1 cup soy milk
1 tablespoon peanut butter
1 tablespoon chia seeds
**1 banana**
**Directions**

In a blender place all ingredients and blend until smooth
Pour smoothie in a glass and serve
**Nutrition:**
calories 321 fat 17
fiber 1.2
carbs 4.4

## 102. Green Juice Smoothie
**Preparation Time: 10 minutes**
**Cooking Time: 0 minutes**
**Servings: 1**
**Ingredients**
**2 apples**
2 celery sticks
**1 cucumber**
1/2 cup kale leaves
**1/4 lemon**
**Directions**
In a blender place all ingredients and blend until smooth
Pour smoothie in a glass and serve
**Nutrition:**
Calories 140
Fat 1 g
Carbohydrate 6 g
Protein 6 g

## 103. Coconut Smoothie
**Preparation Time: 10 minutes**
**Cooking Time: 0 minutes**
**Servings: 1**
**Ingredients**
**1 banana**
2 oz. baby spinach
1 cup mango
1/4 tsp jalapeno pepper
1 cup water

**Directions**
In a blender place all ingredients and blend until smooth
Pour smoothie in a glass and serve
**Nutrition:**
calories 136 fat 4.7

fiber 0.6 carbs 7.5
protein 1

## 104. Peach and Kiwi Smoothie

**Preparation Time: 10 minutes**
**Cooking Time: 0 minutes**
**Servings: 1**
**Ingredients**
1 cup plain low fat yogurt
1/2 cup peach chunks
1 tablespoon protein powder
Water as needed
1/2 cup kiwi fruit

**Directions**
Blend powder and fruits finely in liquid, serve chilled when smooth.
**Nutrition:**
calories 224
fat 1.1
fiber 5.5
carbs 16.7
protein 1

## 105. Smoothie With a Spirit

**Preparation Time: 10 minutes**
**Cooking Time: 0 minutes**
**Servings: 1**
**Ingredients**
1/4 cup greek yogurt
1/2 of a banana
1 teaspoon spirulina
1/4 cup blueberries
1/2 cup chilled almond milk
1/4 cup peach chunks
**Directions**
Mix all the ingredients in a mixing blender and serve as soon as it becomes smooth.
**Nutrition:**
Calories 69
Fat 6.5 g
Fiber 2.6 g
Carbs 10.6 g

Protein 9.4 g

## 106. Smoothie with Ginger and Cucumber

**Preparation Time: 10 minutes**
**Cooking Time: 0 minutes**
**Servings: 1**
**Ingredients**
1 cup chilled water
2 slices of cucumber
1 tablespoon lime juice
Couple of mint leaves
1 small piece of ginger fresh
**Directions**
Add chilled cup of water in an electric mixer, grate ginger piece. Mix with cucumber slices, lime juice and mint leaves to serve.
**Nutrition:**
Calories 170
Fat 3 Fiber 6
Carbs 8 Protein 5

## 107. Buttery Banana Shake

**Preparation Time: 10 minutes**
**Cooking Time: 0 minutes**
**Servings: 1**
**Ingredients**
1 tablespoon raw peanut butter
1 cup almond milk
1 scoop protein powder any flavor
1/4 cup greek yogurt
1 teaspoon basil
1 teaspoon ginger paste
1 teaspoon vanilla extract
1 teaspoon sesame seeds
**Directions**
Mix and blend all ingredients in a blender and shake for a whole minute to drink a smooth shake in the morning or evening during workouts.
**Nutrition:**
Calories 170
Fat 3
Fiber 6

Carbs 8
Protein 5

## 108. Grapefruit Smoothie with cinnamon

**Preparation Time: 10 minutes**
**Cooking Time: 0 minutes**
**Servings: 1**
**Ingredients**
1 cup grapefruit juice, use pulp for fiber (optional)
Ice cubes in crushed form as needed (2-3)
1 cinnamon stick
1 sliced banana
1 teaspoon brown sugar
**Directions**
Mix all ingredients in a blender and mix for 30 seconds to blend well, when done, serve
**Nutrition:**
Calories 170
Fat 3
Fiber 6
Carbs 8
Protein 5

## 109. Melon and Nuts Smoothie

**Preparation Time: 10 minutes**
**Cooking Time: 0 minutes**
**Servings: 1**
**Ingredients**
1 cup water melon chunks
1/4 cup mixed nuts
1 cup soy milk
1/2 cup tofu
Chilled water as needed
1 scoop of chocolate whey protein powder
**Directions**
Blend all ingredients greatly to attain a smooth and soft drink.
**Nutrition:**
Calories 191 Fat 10 Fiber 3

Carbs 13
Protein 1

## 110. Heavy Metal Cleansing Smoothie

**Preparation Time: 10 minutes**
**Cooking Time: 0 minutes**
**Servings: 1**
**Ingredients**
1 cup soy milk
A pinch of turmeric
A pinch of freshly crushed ginger
1 teaspoon cinnamon powder
1 tablespoon maple syrup
A big date without pit
**Directions**
Take a blender and combine all ingredients to mix and serve when smooth. Serve at room temperature or slightly warm as you like.
**Nutrition:**
Calories 69 Fat 6.5 g
Fiber 2.6 g Carbs 10.6 g Protein 9.4 g

## 111. Triple C Shake

**Preparation Time: 10 minutes**
**Cooking Time: 0 minutes**
**Servings: 1**
**Ingredients**
1/4 cup raw spinach
1 tablespoon cacao nibs
1 cup skimmed chocolate nut milk
3/4 cup black or blue berries
A dash of red pepper flakes
A scoop of chocolate whey powder
Water as needed
6 crushed ice cubes
A handful of nuts
A pinch of cinnamon powder
**Directions**
Put all the ingredients in a blender and shake well till smooth. Serve chilled in a large glass and enjoy.
**Nutrition:**
Calories 476 Fat 40

Fiber 9 Carbs 33
Protein 6

# CHAPTER 12:

# Lunch Recipes

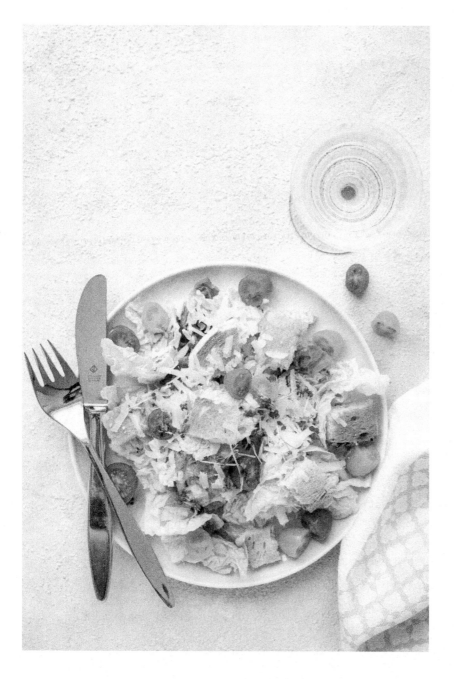

## 112. Vegetarian Fried Chorizo with Chick Peas and Tomatoes

**Preparation Time: 15 Minutes**
**Cooking Time:** 25 Minutes
**Servings: 3**
**Ingredients:**
Salt and pepper
3 tablespoons parsley
2 pints' cherry tomatoes
1 teaspoon smoked paprika
9 ounces' chorizo
2 15oz. cans chickpeas
1 onion
1 tablespoon olive oil
**Directions:**
In a saucepan over medium heat, steam the oil.
Sauté onion for three minutes, or until soft.
Toss in the chorizo.
Sauté for 30 seconds to 1 minute, or until thoroughly hot.
Combine chickpeas, grape tomatoes, and paprika in a mixing bowl.
Cook for 8 minutes, or until tomatoes are softened and liquids are boiling.
Salt and pepper to taste. Serve with a tarragon garnish.
**Nutrition:**
Calories: 344  Carbs: 9
Protein: 28
Total Fat: 17

## 113. Mediterranean Spanish Roasted Vegetables

**Preparation Time: 15 Minutes**
**Cooking Time:** 25 Minutes
**Servings: 3**
**Ingredients:**
Parmesan cheese
Crushed red pepper
1 teaspoon dried thyme
Salt and pepper
8 oz. baby Bella mushrooms
Extra virgin olive oil
1/2 tablespoon dried oregano
12 oz. baby potatoes
2 zucchini or summer squash
12 large garlic cloves
12 oz. Campari tomatoes
**Directions:**
Preheat the oven to 375 degrees Fahrenheit.
In a big mixing bowl, combine the mushrooms, vegetables, and garlic.
Drizzle a generous amount of olive oil on top.
Insert the sesame oil, tarragon, salt, and pepper to taste. Toss all together.
Take just the potatoes and lay them out on a baking pan that has been lightly greased.
Roast for ten minutes in a preheated oven.
Remove the pan from the heat and add half veggies and mushrooms.
Return to the oven for a final 20 minutes of roasting or until the vegetables are forktender.
Mix thoroughly with smashed cayenne pepper and chopped fresh Parmesan cheese.
**Nutrition:**
Calories: 207  Carbs: 7.8
Protein: 29.5  Total Fat: 6.8

## 114. Tapas & Pinchos Vegetarian

**Preparation Time: 15 Minutes**
**Cooking Time:** 25 Minutes
**Servings: 3**
**Ingredients:**
**Garlic Aioli Ingredients**
1/2 cup olive oil
Salt to taste
1 teaspoon lemon juice
1 egg yolk
1 garlic clove

**Tomato Sauce Ingredients**

2 teaspoons smoked paprika

Salt and pepper to taste

1 garlic clove

1 red jalapeno

1 tablespoon olive oil

3 large plum tomatoes

**Potato Ingredients**

2 tablespoons olive oil

Salt and pepper to taste

1 lb. potatoes

Garnish Ingredients

Fresh lemon juice

1 tablespoon parsley

**Directions:**

Preheat the oven to 400 degrees Fahrenheit.

Toss potato in canola oil and season with salt and pepper.

Position on a cookie sheet in a single sheet.

Cook for 25 to 30 minutes until its fork ready.

In a spice grinder, puree the vegetables to make the sauce.

Add the oil to a pan.

Garlic and jalapeno peppers should be added at this stage.

Insert pureed onions, cayenne pepper, salt, and pepper until the onions have softened.

Combine the garlic, lime juice, and egg white in a mixing dish.

Beat the egg yolks with an immersion blender until they are light in color.

Continue to beat until it thickens into a sour cream texture.

Mix in the salt until it is well combined.

Put potatoes in a dish to eat.

**Nutrition:**

Calories: 336 Carbs: 1

Protein: 56

Total Fat: 10

# 115. Vegetarian Spanish Toast with Escalivada

**Preparation Time: 15 Minutes**

**Cooking Time:** 25 Minutes

**Servings: 3**

**Ingredients:**

Flatleaf parsley

Sea salt

80g soft goat's cheese

1 slice Serrano ham

1/2 jar of Escalivada

Green olives

Extra virgin olive oil

1 large bruschetta bread

**Directions:**

After toasting one side of the bruschetta crust, sprinkle the uncooked side with olive oil.

Drain the escalivada with a fork.

Place the whole or doubled olives on top, then sprinkle the goat's cheese on top.

Put the toast back under the flame.

Blow the Spicy salami into small pieces and sprinkle them on top.

Cut into chunks or half and serve hot with a side dish of finely chopped flatleaf parsley and sea salt pinch.

**Nutrition:**

Calories: 333

Carbs: 8.9

Protein: 60.6

Total Fat: 4.7

# 116. Vegetarian Garlic Soup with Egg and Croutons

**Preparation Time: 15 Minutes**

**Cooking Time:** 25 Minutes

**Servings: 3**

**Ingredients:**

1/4 cup extra virgin olive oil

Salt and pepper

1 teaspoon sweet paprika

1liter chicken broth

2 eggs
6 garlic cloves
2 slices of stale bread
**Directions:**
Garlic should be peeled and cut into strips.
Heat the olive oil in a saucepan over medium heat.
Add garlic and cook for 23 minutes, or until it starts to brown.
Add the loaf to the pan and fry it with the garlic, allowing it to soak up the oil.
Reduce to low heat and stir in the parmesan.
Put in the liquid and give it a good swirl.
Take the soup to a rolling simmer, reduce to low heat, and continue cooking for about thirty minutes.
To taste, season with salt and pepper, using at least 1/2 teaspoon pepper.
In a large mixing bowl, whisk together the eggs and add them to the soup.
**Nutrition:**
Calories: 420
Carbs: 16
Protein: 30
Total Fat: 26

# 117. Mediterranean Baked Vegetarian Tapas
**Preparation Time: 15 Minutes**
**Cooking Time:** 25 Minutes
**Servings: 3**
**Ingredients:**
1 tablespoon olive oil
Fresh basil
1 red onion
1 dl mató cheese
1 bag of dates
250g small tomatoes
2 clove of garlic
2 tablespoon mató cheese
A handful walnuts
1 eggplant

1 tablespoon maple syrup
**Directions:**
Roll the dates and fill them with hazelnuts and Spanish Mató cheese.
Place on a tray and drizzle with maple syrup to finish.
Wash the tomatoes and cut them in half.
Parsley and red onion should be chopped.
Combine the tomato and Mató cheese in a mixing dish.
Wash the eggplant and break it into thin slices.
Steam for 23 minutes on each side after brushing with canola oil.
Cover them in foil and place them on a tray.
Place olive tapenade, polenta, cello, oranges, artichokes, manchego cheese, heat tomatoes, fluffy biscuits, and Spanish wine on the tapas table.
**Nutrition:**
Calories: 294
Carbs: 11
Protein: 23.9
Total Fat: 18.2

# 118. Vegetarian Pan con Tomate
**Preparation Time: 15 Minutes**
**Cooking Time:** 25 Minutes
**Servings: 3**
**Ingredients:**
2 medium cloves garlic
Flaky sea salt
1 loaf ciabatta
Extravirgin olive oil
Kosher salt
2 large tomatoes
**Directions:**
Tomatoes should be cut in half vertically. In a big mixing bowl, grate a box grinder.

Preheat the broiler to high and position the rack four inches below it.

Spoonful olive oil over the cut side of the bread on a work surface.

Use kosher salt, season to taste.

Position the bread cutting side up on a rack set in a pan or immediately on the griddle rack and broil for two or three minutes, or until crispy and beginning to char form around the edge.

Take the bread from the microwave and scrub it with the garlic cloves that have been cut.

Spread the tomato mixture on top of the pizza.

Dress with flaky sesame oil and rain of extravirgin canola oil.

**Nutrition:**
Calories: 251
Carbs: 1
Protein: 34
Total Fat: 12

## 119. Vegetarian Spanish Mixed Green Salad

**Preparation Time: 15 Minutes**
**Cooking Time:** 25 Minutes
**Servings: 3**
**Ingredients:**
1/2 Spanish onion
10 12 green olives
2 cups Boston lettuce
2 tomatoes
1 cup baby spinach
2 cups romaine lettuce
Dressing
3 tablespoons olive oil
Sea salt and black pepper
1 tablespoon lemon juice
**Directions:**
Combine all of the dressing components in a mixing bowl and whisk until thoroughly combined.
Toss with salad well before eating.
**Nutrition:**

Calories: 240 Carbs: 16
Protein: 25  Total Fat: 8

## 120. Vegetarian Spanish Rice Dinner

**Preparation Time: 15 Minutes**
**Cooking Time:** 25 Minutes
**Servings: 3**
**Ingredients:**
1/8 teaspoon pepper
1/8 teaspoon hot pepper sauce
1/2 teaspoon ground mustard
1/4 teaspoon garlic powder
1 teaspoon salt
1 teaspoon Worcestershire sauce
1 tablespoon onion
1 tablespoon sugar
1 can stewed tomatoes
1 can green beans
11/2 cups cooked rice
1 pound ground beef
**Directions:**
Steam beef when no pinker in a large frying pan; clean.
Add the rest of the ingredients and stir to combine.
Raise the temperature to be high and bring the mixture to a boil.
Reduce to a low heat environment, cover, and cook for 510 minutes, or until thoroughly cooked.
**Nutrition:**
Calories: 282
Carbs: 8.2
Protein: 24.4
Total Fat: 15.4

## 121. Champinones Spanish Garlic Mushrooms

**Preparation Time: 15 Minutes**
**Cooking Time:** 25 Minutes
**Servings: 3**
**Ingredients:**
1 tablespoon lemon juice
2 tablespoons fresh parsley

Salt to taste
1/2 cup white wine
4 garlic cloves
2 pounds' mushrooms
2 tablespoons olive oil
**Directions:**
In a large skillet over medium heat, add the oil over moderate flame.
Cook the mushroom for five minutes, periodically tossing the pot.
Heat, flipping the pan often, for another 12 minutes or until crispy, adding the garlic, cayenne pepper, salt, and pepper.
Toss in the tarragon to mix everything.
Aioli and lime wedges should be served alongside the mushrooms.
**Nutrition:**
Calories: 284
Carbs: 1.4
Protein: 24.2
Total Fat: 17

## 122. Greek Vegetarian Stuffed Zucchini

**Preparation Time: 15 Minutes**
**Cooking Time:** 25 Minutes
**Servings: 3**
**Ingredients:**
8 pitted Kalamata olives
1/2 cup crumbled feta cheese
1 cup cooked quinoa
1 cup diced plum tomatoes
4 medium zucchini
3/4 teaspoon smoked paprika
1 tablespoon chopped fresh oregano
3/4 cup chopped onion
1 tablespoon garlic
1/4 teaspoon salt
1 tablespoon extravirgin olive oil
1/2 teaspoon ground pepper
**Directions:**
Heat the oven to 350 degrees F.
Break each zucchini in quarter lengthwise, use a fork, scrape much of the skin, preserving 1/2inchthick cores.

Chop quarter the flesh thinly sliced; waste the remainder flesh or save it for some purpose.
Cover a baking dish with the zucchini pellets; brush with salt and black pepper.
Bake for 15 to 20 minutes before the zucchini begins to soften.
In the meantime, over a moderate flame, heat the oil in a large skillet.
Add the sliced zucchini, onions, cloves, paprika, and two tablespoons of oregano; boil for approximately 3 minutes, stirring regularly, until the onion begins to soften.
Stir in the quinoa, olives, tomatoes, and feta, and extract from the heat.
Split the zucchini cores equally.
Turn to broil the oven and put a rack 8 inches away from the heat.
Broil the cores of packed zucchini till the edges are finely browned for four to six minutes.
Stir with 1 teaspoon of the leftover oregano.
**Nutrition:**
Calories: 217
Carbs: 16.7
Protein: 25.5
Total Fat: 6.3

## 123. Greek Vegetarian Soutzoukakia

**Preparation Time: 15 Minutes**
**Cooking Time:** 25 Minutes
**Servings: 3**
**Ingredients:**
**For the Oriental Meatballs**
Pepper
200g allpurpose flour
1 tablespoon parsley
Salt
500g chickpeas

1 clove of garlic
1 bunch mint
3 tablespoon olive oil
lemon juice, of 1/2 lemon
3 onions, dry
1 teaspoon cumin, powder
lemon zest, of 1 lemon
1 tablespoon baking powder
**For the Sauce**
Salt
Pepper
1 tablespoon tomato paste
3 tomatoes
1 clove of garlic
1 teaspoon granulated sugar
2 tablespoon olive oil
1 teaspoon oregano
1 chili pepper, dried
1 onion, dry
3 bay leaves
1 stick cinnamon
**Directions:**
Put a reasonable quantity of water in a jar with the chickpeas and continue cooking.
Wash them before they break for twelve hours or overnight.
Dump, washed off when prepared.
Move and pulse a bit to a mixing bowl, ensuring you do not produce a paste.
Put the olive oil, baking soda, cilantro, lime zest, lime juice, diced onion, grated cloves, coarsely chopped mint, salt, and black pepper in a bowl transfer to the mixture. Rigorously blend.
Form the combination into ovalshaped meatballs and excavate in the starch.
Over moderate to low heat, put a large pan and heat the oil let it get heated. Insert the meatballs cautiously in quantities and cook until they become golden.

To drain, switch to a cooking pan filled with paper towels.
Put the olive oil, the finely diced onion, the bay leaf, the spices, the dried oregano, the mustard, the hot pepper, the crushed garlic cloves, the granulated sugar, and the tomato sauce in a shallow bowl.
Garnish with the grated onion, salt, and black pepper.
Reduce the heat and add the crispy meatballs to the dish. Cover and cook with a cap for ten minutes.
Present with boiling basmati rice, rosemary, canola oil, and clean oregano.
**Nutrition:**
Calories: 371
Carbs: 1.7
Protein: 33.7
Total Fat: 25.1

## 124. Greek Steamed Vegetable Bowls
**Preparation Time: 15 Minutes**
**Cooking Time:** 25 Minutes
**Servings: 3**
**Ingredients:**
**For the Steamed Vegetables**
Olive oil
Salt and black pepper
2 medium bell peppers
8 ounces mushrooms
2 medium zucchini
1 red onion
**For the Bowls**
Salt and black pepper
Pita chips
Fresh dill and basil
Avocado Tzatziki
2 cups cooked farro
1/2 cup Kalamata olives
1/2 cup crumbled feta cheese
15 oz. chickpeas
1 cup halved grape tomatoes
1 cucumber

## For the Lemon Dressing

1 teaspoon dried oregano
Kosher salt and black pepper
1/2 teaspoon Dijon mustard
2 cloves garlic
1/2 cup olive oil
2 tablespoons lemon juice
1/2 cup red wine vinegar

**Directions:**

Heat the Steam to high.
Sprinkle with olive oil over the veggies and add salt and pepper.
Roast the veggies until crispy and Steam marks emerge, flipping once.
Take it from the fire.
Mix the olive oil, Dijon mustard, white wine vinegar, lime juice, cloves, oregano, pepper, and salt in a shallow saucepan or container to make the coating.
Thinly slice the roasted veggies to fill the bowls.
Cover each dish with the Steamed peppers, cucumber, chickpeas, Kalamata olives, tomatoes, and feta cheese and split the farro into 4 cups.
Garnish with spices and, to taste, sprinkle with salt. Sprinkle and eat with tzatziki and pita chips with seasoning.

**Nutrition:**

Calories: 385
Carbs: 48.5
Protein: 24.5
Total Fat: 8.5

## 125. reek Veggie Balls With Tahini Lemon Sauce

**Preparation Time: 15 Minutes**
**Cooking Time:** 25 Minutes
**Servings: 3**
**Ingredients:**

1 large lemon
2 15ounce cans of blackeyed peas
1/2 cup whole wheat breadcrumbs
1/2 cup nut meal

1 medium red onion
Pinch sea salt
1/4 cup ground flax seeds
3 cloves garlic
1 tablespoon oregano
1/2 teaspoon black pepper
5 soft dates
1/2 cup fresh parsley
1 teaspoon fennel seeds
1/4 cup sliced sundried tomatoes
Tahini Lemon Sauce
Water
Smoked paprika
2 cloves garlic
1/4 teaspoon black pepper
1 large lemon
1/2 cup tahini

**Directions:**

Position the spring onions, parsley, cloves, oregano, sundried tomatoes, dates, fennel seeds, salt, and black pepper in the spice grinder bag. Work until finely chopped.
In the food processor, add the flax seeds, cornflour, almond flour, and lime juice and pulse until mixed.
Insert the blackeyed pods into the food processor till the beans are crushed, though not purified, for a few seconds.
Take the mixture out of the food processor and cool it for thirty minutes.

In the meantime, mix all the tahini with lime juice, cloves, and black pepper to create Tahini Citrus Sauce.
Add more water, according to the ideal consistency, to form a delicious sauce.
Spray with paprika, which has been smoked.
Preheat the furnace to 375 F.
Use your palms to roll vegetarian balls into 24 golfsized balls, and put them on a cookie dish coated with cooking

spray. Position it on the oven's topshelf.

Cook for 60 minutes, until the vegetarian balls are baked, and the surface is lightly browned.

Use Tahini Citrus Sauce to serve.

**Nutrition:**
Calories: 433  Carbs: 10
Protein: 38 Total Fat: 26

## 126. Vegetarian Greek Mpougiourdi

**Preparation Time: 15 Minutes**
**Cooking Time:** 25 Minutes
**Servings: 3**
**Ingredients:**
1 pinch oregano
1 splash olive oil
1/2 green hot pepper
1/2 sliced tomato
1 slice yellow cheese
1 slice Greek feta cheese

**Directions:**
Cut the tomatoes and the spice pepper. Put the feta cheese in an ovensafe dish and then cover that with some sliced tomatoes and some chili pepper.

Close and cover again with tomato and chili pepper with a strong melted yellow cheese.

Add a little canola oil and a dash of oregano to the mixture.

Toast for ten minutes in a preheated oven or two minutes on the stove.

**Nutrition:**
Calories: 453
Carbs: 20
Protein: 28
Total Fat: 46

## 127. Brian Greek Roasted Vegetables

**Preparation Time: 15 Minutes**
**Cooking Time:** 25 Minutes
**Servings: 3**

**Ingredients:**
1 can diced tomatoes
3 sprigs thyme
1/2 teaspoon salt
1/4 teaspoon ground black pepper
1 large potato
1 cloves garlic minced
1 large tomato
1/2 cup extravirgin olive oil
1 teaspoon oregano
1 zucchini
1 red onion
1 eggplant

**Directions:**
Begin with the veggies getting cut.

For slicing through circular forms, you can either choose a mandolin cutter or a razor blade.

To make a lovely Briam and vegetables to bake uniformly, try to choose veggies identical in volume.

Add the cut vegetables to a big bowl and stir and rain with the vegetable oil.

Add the oregano, garlic, pepper, and salt.

Give a decent mix to all so that the vegetables are prepared well.

Add the tomato sauce and 1/2 cup of water to an ovenproof pan. Then organize, in lines, the seasoned veggies.

In the blending cup, if there is any coconut oil remaining, pour it over the veggies.

Mold the baking sheet with foil and put it in an oven, and bake.

Cook for thirty minutes at 390°F (200°C), test if the vegetables are tender, and cover the foil.

Roast for another 1020 minutes to minimize the fluid and the veggies get their golden brown hue.

To get the vegetables to caramelize a little, you might want to put the dish underneath the Steam for five minutes.

Serve with olives, feta cheese, and moldy rolls.

**Nutrition:**
Calories: 117
Carbs: 5.8
Protein: 13.9
Total Fat: 3.7

## 128. Yemista (Stuffed Peppers and Tomatoes)

**Preparation Time:** 15 Minutes
**Cooking Time:** 25 Minutes
**Servings:** 3
**Ingredients:**

- 4 potatoes
1/2 cup toasted breadcrumbs
1/2 cup olive oil
Salt and pepper
2 tablespoons tomato paste
1 teaspoon cinnamon
1/2 cup parsley
1 tablespoon dried oregano
4 large tomatoes
1/4 cup fresh mint
3 cloves of garlic
1/2 cup lean mince
1 medium onion
4 large red peppers

**Directions:**
Heat the oven to 180C.
Trim the ends off between 12 cm from the edge of the tomatoes and peppers.
Strip the juice from the tomatoes and peppers.
Slice the onions.
Finely cut the cloves and sauté this in a bowl with onions.
Transfer the pulp as well as the other spices and herbs from the tomato.
Add the paste of tomatoes.
Cover the solution with the veggies and swap the tops.
With the roasted potatoes, cover the veggies.
Sprinkle with oil appropriately.
Spray with breadcrumbs and end with salt and black pepper.
Cook for 1 hour in the oven.

**Nutrition:**
Calories: 268
Carbs: 12.6
Protein: 41.7

## 129. Greek Vegetarian Meatballs

**Preparation Time:** 15 Minutes
**Cooking Time:** 25 Minutes
**Servings:** 3
**Ingredients:**
2 tablespoon tahini
3 tablespoon mixture of parsley, mint, and dill
2 1/2 teaspoon fresh oregano
1/2 teaspoon red pepper flake
1 cup Quinoa
1/2 cup diced shallot
Salt and pepper to taste
4 tablespoon olive oil
3 cloves garlic
1 15oz. can black beans

**Directions:**
Heat the oven to 350 °F.
On a parchmentlined baking tray, position the dry kidney beans and cook for 1015 minutes till the beans look broken and sound dry to the touch.
Take them from the furnace and raise the heat of the oven to 370°F.
Over mediumhigh heat, heat a large pan.
Add two tablespoons of olive oil, cloves, and parsley once it is warmed.
Sauté for three minutes, or until transparent and moderately soft, stirring regularly.
For later usage, remove from the heat and reserve the bowl.
In a mixing bowl, add kidney beans alongside cloves, parsley, salt, black pepper, pepper flake, oregano, and process a few times into a slim meal, becoming cautious not to mix thoroughly.
When squeezed between your fingertips, insert the quinoa, rice, tahini, chopped parsley, basil, dill, and rotate to mix until a contoured dough shape.

Add a little more starch and shake to mix, whether it is too tacky or muddy.

Squeeze out heaping volumes of 11 1/2 tablespoon and shape carefully using your palms into tiny pieces.

Patting these first and tossing them afterward. Place in a dish and chill in the fridge for fifteen minutes.

Chilling is acceptable, but during skillet frying, it means the meatball holds together longer.

In a small container, put the remaining 1/4 of a cup of starch.

Reheat the pan and transfer the remaining olive oil to the pan.

Brush the meatballs with powder and return them to the skillet and sauté for a few minutes, rotating the meatballs slightly to either surface to get a soft crust.

Then move to the oven and cook for 20 minutes or until the sides are nicely browned and gently dry to the fingertips.

**Nutrition:**
Calories: 258  Carbs: 7.3
Protein: 28  Total Fat: 13.4

## 130. Greek Goddess Bowl
**Preparation Time: 15 Minutes**
**Cooking Time:** 25 Minutes
**Servings: 3**
**Ingredients:**
Chickpeas
1 tablespoon maple syrup
1/4 teaspoon sea salt
1 tablespoon shawarma spice blend
1 tablespoon oil
1 15ounce can chickpeas
Bowl
1 medium cucumber
1 medium carrot
3/4 cup Vegan Tzatziki
1/2 cup Kalamata olives
1/2 cup cherry tomatoes

1 batch red pepper
**For serving**
Garlic Dill Sauce
Tahini Dressing
Traditional Vegan Falafel
Vegan Flatbread or Naan
**Directions:**
Heat the oven to 190C and placed a baking sheet in place.

Alongside oil, shawarma seasoning blend, golden syrup, and salt, apply clean chickpeas to a blending cup. To mix, flip.

To the baking dish, add the prepared chickpeas.

Toast for 23 minutes or until lightly browned and the chickpeas are somewhat crispy. Take it out of the oven and set it aside.

Divide the tzatziki, onions, tabbouleh, cucumber, olives, and vegetables (optional) into two serving bowls to complete the dish.

Cover with cooked chickpeas and add fresh lime juice to garnish.

However, better when new, you can store leftover food in the fridge for up to 34 days.

Place the remaining chickpeas individually in a sealed jar for up to 3 days at ambient temperature or up to one month in the refrigerator.

## 131. Greek LasagnaVegetarian
**Preparation Time: 15 Minutes**
**Cooking Time:** 25 Minutes
**Servings: 3**
**Ingredients:**
**Tomato Sauce**
1/2 teaspoon black pepper
3 tablespoons dill
1/2 cup chopped Kalamata olive
2 teaspoons salt
3 tablespoons olive oil

2 teaspoons marjoram, dried
5 cups tomatoes
5 garlic cloves, minced
2 cups chopped onions

**Filling**
3 cups grated feta cheese
1/2 lb. uncooked lasagna noodle
2 cups of cottage cheese
1 teaspoon ground fennel
Olive oil, for brushing
3 eggs, beaten
1 large eggplant

**Directions:**
Heat the oil slightly over mediumhigh heat in a frying pan.

Insert the onions and sauté for about five minutes, stirring regularly before the liquids have started to come out of the onions.

Mix in the cloves and marjoram till the onions are transparent, and sauté.

Insert the tomatoes, cover them, and get them to a boil. Then reduce the flame, only enough to hold a spot, to moderate low.

Olives, pepper, and salt are added. Before preparing the lasagna for the perfect taste, insert the dill.

Preheat a 400F furnace. Oil the broad baking sheet gently.

Place the eggplant circles on a baking tray as the sauce softly simmers—brush olive oil on them.

Cook for about fifteen minutes, exposed.

Replace the oven's eggplant and turn the heat down to 350F.

In the meantime, blend all the eggs, fennel, cottage cheese, and 1 cup feta cheese in a bowl and whisk.

**Nutrition:**
Calories: 257
Carbs: 10
Protein: 29

Total Fat: 10

## 132. GreekStyle Baked Feta Recipe

**Preparation Time: 15 Minutes**
**Cooking Time:** 25 Minutes
**Servings: 3**
**Ingredients:**
Fresh mint leaves
Crusty bread
Extravirgin olive oil
8 oz. feta cheese
1/2 teaspoon red pepper flakes
4 fresh thyme sprigs
1/2 cup cherry tomatoes
2 teaspoon oregano
1/2 red onion
1/2 green bell pepper

**Directions:**
Preheat oven to 400 degrees F and modify a tray in the center.

Organize the onions, green peppers, and grape tomatoes at the lower part of a ramekin or stove dish.

Spray some of the new thyme with 1 teaspoon oregano, chili flakes, and apply most of it. Drizzle some extravirgin olive oil with it.

On top of the prepared vegetables, add the feta.

Prepare the leftover dried oregano with both the feta cube, a touch of chili flakes, and whatever is left of the fresh thyme.

Sprinkle the feta with a thick layer of olive oil and ensure to rub some of the butter on the edges.

Position the baking sheet on the oven's center rack and bake for 20 minutes.

Serve it with tortilla chips or Spanish toasted bread.

**Nutrition:**
Calories: 152
Carbs: 2
Protein: 6

Total Fat: 14

## 133. Chicken Stir Fry

**Preparation Time: 15 Minutes**
**Cooking Time:** 25 Minutes
**Servings: 3**
**Ingredients:**
1/2 cup chicken broth, low sodium
12 ounces skinless chicken breasts, cut into strips
1 cup red bell pepper, seeded and chopped
8 ounces (1 cup) broccoli, cut into florets
1 teaspoon crushed red pepper
**Directions:**
Place a small amount of chicken broth in a saucepan. Heat over medium flame and stir in the chicken. Water sautés the chicken for at least 5 minutes while stirring constantly.
Place the rest of the ingredients and stir.
Cover the pan with lid and cook for another 5 minutes.
**Nutrition:**
Calories per serving: 137
Protein: 15g
Carbs: 15.4g
Fat: 1.2g
Sugar: 0.6g

## 134. Lean and Green Garlic Chicken with Zoodles

**Preparation Time: 15 Minutes**
**Cooking Time:** 25 Minutes
**Servings: 3**
**Ingredients:**
1 1/2 pounds boneless and skinless chicken breasts, cut into bitesized pieces
6 slices sundried tomatoes
1 teaspoon chopped garlic
1 cup low fat plain Greek yogurt
1/2 cup chicken broth, low sodium
1/2 teaspoon garlic powder
1/2 teaspoon Italian seasoning
1 cup spinach, chopped
1 1/2 cup zucchini, cut into thin noodles
**Directions:**
Place 2 tablespoons water in a pan and heat over lowmedium flame.
Water sautés the chicken for 3 minutes while stirring constantly until the sides are slightly golden.
Stir in the tomatoes and garlic and stir for another 3 minutes. Add in the yogurt, chicken broth, garlic powder, and Italian seasoning.
Cover with lid and allow simmering for at least 7 minutes.
Stir in the spinach last. Cook for another 2 minutes.
Place the zucchini noodles in a deep dish and pour over the chicken. Toss the noodles to coat with the sauce.
Serve immediately.
**Nutrition:**
Calories per serving: 205
Protein: 33.3g
Carbs: 6g
Fat: 2g
Sugar: 1.2g

## 135. Lean and Green "Macaroni

**Preparation Time: 15 Minutes**
**Cooking Time:** 25 Minutes
**Servings: 3**
**Ingredients:**
2 tablespoons yellow onion, diced
5 ounces 9597% lean ground beef
2 tablespoons light thousand island dressing
1/8 teaspoon apple cider vinegar
1/8 teaspoon onion powder
3 cups Romaine lettuce, shredded
2 tablespoons lowfat cheddar cheese, shredded

1ounce dill pickle slices
1 teaspoon sesame seeds

**Directions:**

Put 3 tablespoons of water in a pan and heat over mediumlow flame. Water sauté the onions for 30 seconds before adding the beef. Sauté the beef for 4 minutes while stirring constantly.

Add in the Thousand Island dressing, apple cider vinegar, and onion powder. Close the lid and keep on cooking for 5 minutes. Remove the lid and allow simmering until the sauce thickens. Turn off the heat and allow the beef to rest and cool.

In a bowl, place the lettuce at the bottom and pour in the beef. Layer with cheddar cheese, and pickles. Sprinkle with sesame on top.

**Nutrition:**

Calories per serving: 119
Protein: 10.8g
Carbs: 4.4g
Fat: 2.1g
Sugar: 2.5g

## 136. Lean and Green Broccoli Taco

**Preparation Time: 15 Minutes**
**Cooking Time:** 25 Minutes
**Servings: 3**
**Ingredients:**
4 ounces 9597% lean ground beef
1/4 cup roma tomatoes, chopped
1/4 teaspoon garlic powder
1/4 teaspoon onion powder
1 1/4 cup broccoli, cut into bitesized pieces
A pinch of red pepper flakes
1 ounce lowsodium cheddar cheese, shredded ?

**Directions:**

Place 3 tablespoons of water in a pan and heat over medium flame. Water sauté the beef and tomatoes for 5 minutes until the tomatoes are wilted.

Add in the garlic and onion powder and stir for another 3 minutes.

Add the broccoli and close the lid. Cook for another 5 minutes.

Garnish with red pepper flakes and cheddar cheese on top.

**Nutrition:**

Calories per serving: 97
Protein: 9.9 g
Carbs: 2.6g
Fat: 1.7g
Sugar: 0.9 g

## 137. Lean and Green Crunchy Chicken Tacos

**Preparation Time: 15 Minutes**
**Cooking Time:** 25 Minutes
**Servings: 3**
**Ingredients:**
1/2 cup low sodium chicken stock
2 chicken breasts, minced
1 red onion, chopped
1 clove of garlic, minced
3 plum tomatoes, chopped
1 teaspoon cumin powder
1 teaspoon cinnamon powder
1 teaspoon ground coriander
1 red onion, chopped
1/2 red chili, chopped
1 tablespoon lime juice
Meat from 1 ripe avocado
1 cucumber, sliced into thick rounds

**Directions:**

Place a tablespoon of chicken stock in a pan and heat over medium flame. Water sauté the chicken, onion, garlic, and tomatoes for 4 minutes or until the tomatoes have wilted.

Season with cumin, cinnamon, and coriander. Reduce the heat to low and cook for another 5 minutes. Set aside and allow cooling.

In a bowl, mix together the onion, chili, lime juice, and mashed avocado. This is the salsa.

Scoop the salsa and top on sliced cucumber. Top with cooked chicken.

**Nutrition:**
Calories per serving: 313
Protein: 31.8g
Carbs: 14.9 g
Fat: 3.8g
Sugar: 5g

## 138. Cauliflower with Kale Pesto

**Preparation Time: 15 Minutes**
**Cooking Time:** 25 Minutes
**Servings: 3**
**Ingredients:**
3 cups cauliflower, cut into florets
3 cups raw kale, stems removed
2 cups fresh basil
2 tablespoons extra virgin olive oil
3 tablespoons lemon juice
3 cloves of garlic
1/4 teaspoon salt

**Directions:**
Put enough water in a pot and bring to a boil over medium flame. Blanch the cauliflower for 2 minutes. Drain then place in a bowl of icecold water for 5 minutes. Drain again.
In a blender, add the rest of the ingredients. Pulse until smooth.
Pour over the pesto over the cooked cauliflower.

**Nutrition:**
Calories per serving: 41
Protein: 1.8g Carbs: 5g
Fat: 5.3g Sugar: 1.4g

## 139. Lean and Green Chicken Chili

**Preparation Time: 15 Minutes**
**Cooking Time:** 25 Minutes
**Servings: 3**
**Ingredients:**
1pound boneless skinless chicken breast, chopped

1 teaspoon ground cumin
1 cup chopped poblano pepper
1/2 cup chopped onion
1 clove of garlic, minced
2 cups lowsodium chicken broth
1 cup rehydrated pinto beans
1 cup chopped tomatoes
2 tablespoons minced cilantro

**Directions:**
Place all ingredients except the cilantro in a pressure cooker.
Close the lid and set the vent to the sealing position.
Cook on high for 45 minutes until the beans are soft.
Garnish with cilantro before serving

**Nutrition:**
Calories per serving: 229
Protein: 26.1g
Carbs: 23.9g
Fat: 2g Sugar: 2.2g

## 140. Lean and Green Broccoli Alfredo

**Preparation Time: 15 Minutes**
**Cooking Time:** 25 Minutes
**Servings: 3**
**Ingredients:**
2 heads of broccoli, cut into florets
2 tablespoons lemon juice, freshly squeezed
1/2 cup cashew, soaked for 2 hours in water then drained
2 tablespoons white miso, low sodium
2 teaspoon Dijon mustard
Freshly cracked black pepper

**Directions:**
Boil water in a pot over medium flame. Blanch the broccoli for 2 minutes then place in a bowl of iced water. Drain.
In a food processor, place the remaining ingredients and pulse until smooth.

Pour the Alfredo sauce over the broccoli. Toss to coat with the sauce.

**Nutrition:**
Calories per serving: 359
Protein: 10.6g
Carbs: 50.2 g
Fat: 8.4g
Sugar: 2.4g

## 141. Lean and Green Steak Machine

**Preparation Time: 15 Minutes**
**Cooking Time:** 25 Minutes
**Servings: 3**
**Ingredients:**
1/2 teaspoon extra virgin olive oil
2 ounces Sirloin steak, 98% lean
Salt and pepper to taste
1 zucchini, cut into long thin strips
1 onion, chopped
6 ounces asparagus, blanched
4 ounces peas, blanched
**Directions:**
Heat olive oil in a skillet. Season the steak with salt and pepper to taste.
Place in the skillet and sear the steak for 5 minutes on each side. Allow to rest for five minutes before slicing into strips.
Place the remaining ingredients in a bowl and season with salt and pepper to taste  Top with steak strips then toss to combine all ingredients.
**Nutrition:**
Calories per serving: 174
Protein: 4.2g Carbs:  10.3g
 Fat: 4.1g Sugar: 2.1g

## 142. Lean and Green Crockpot Chili

**Preparation Time: 15 Minutes**
**Cooking Time:** 25 Minutes
**Servings: 3**
**Ingredients:**

pound boneless skinless chicken breasts, cut into strips
1/2 cup chopped onion
2 teaspoons ground cumin
1 teaspoon minced garlic
1/2 teaspoon chili powder
Salt and pepper to taste
1 1/2 cups water
1 can green enchilada sauce
1/2 cup dried beans, soaked overnight
**Directions:**
Place all ingredients in a pot.
Mix all ingredients until combined.
Close the lid and turn on the heat to medium.
Bring to a boil and allow to simmer for 45 minutes or until the beans are cooked.
Serve with chopped cilantro on top.
**Nutrition:**
Calories per serving: 84
Protein: 13.4g
Carbs: 3.6 g
Fat: 1.7g
Sugar: 0.8g

## 143. Buffalo Cauliflower Bites

**Preparation Time: 15 Minutes**
**Cooking Time:** 25 Minutes
**Servings: 3**
**Ingredients:**
Cauliflower florets,5 1/2 cup or cooked,4 1/2 cups (9 Greens)
 Buffalo hot sauce, divided,1/2 cup, (4 Condiments)
 Garlic powder,1/4 tsp., (1/2 Condiment)
 Blue cheese or light ranch dressing, divided,6 tbsp., (3 Healthy Fats)
**Directions:**
Put in 1/4 cup of garlic powder and hot buffalo sauce in the cauliflower florets. Toss in order to coat it with the dressing.

For easy cleanup, use cooking spray or put parchment paper (do not use wax paper) on the base of the air fryer. After setting the air fryer to 360, cook for 13 to 15 minutes, stirring every 5 minutes.

In a mediumsize bowl, put the cooked cauliflower and add the excess 1/4 cup of Buffalo Hot Sauce. Coat by tossing. Relish with 2 tbsp. of blue cheese or light ranch dressing!

If using the oven, at 450 degrees, cook for 20 min, mixing when half done.

Nutrition:
(calories): 14
Protein: 1.03
Fat: 0.22 g
Carbohydrates: 2.67 g

## 144. Ravaging Beef Pot Roast

**Preparation Time: 15 Minutes**
**Cooking Time:** 25 Minutes
**Servings: 3**
**Ingredients:**
3 1/2 pounds beef roast
4 ounces mushrooms, sliced
12 ounces beef stock
1ounce onion soup mix
1/2 cup Italian dressing, low sodium, and low fat
**Directions:**
Take a bowl and add the stock, onion soup mix and Italian dressing.
Stir.
Put beef roast in pan.
Add mushrooms, stock mix to the pan and cover with foil.
Preheat your oven to 300 degrees F.
Bake for 1 hour and 15 minutes.
Let the roast cool.
Slice and serve.
Enjoy with the gravy on top!
**Nutrition:**
Calories: 700

Fat: 56g
Carbohydrates: 10g
Protein: 70g

## 145. Lovely Faux Mac and Cheese

**Preparation Time: 15 Minutes**
**Cooking Time:** 25 Minutes
**Servings: 3**
**Ingredients:**
5 cups cauliflower florets
Sunflower seeds and pepper to taste
1 cup coconut almond milk
1/2 cup vegetable broth
2 tablespoons coconut flour, sifted
1 organic egg, beaten
1 cup cashew cheese
**Directions:**
Preheat your oven to 350 degrees F.
Season florets with sunflower seeds and steam until firm.
Place florets in a greased ovenproof dish.
Heat coconut almond milk over medium heat in a skillet, make sure to season the oil with sunflower seeds and pepper.
Stir in broth and add coconut flour to the mix, stir.
Cook until the sauce begins to bubble.
Remove heat and add beaten egg.
Pour the thick sauce over the cauliflower and mix in cheese.
Bake for 3045 minutes.
Serve and enjoy!
**Nutrition:**
Calories: 229
Fat: 14g
Carbohydrates: 9g
Protein: 15g

## 146. Epic Mango Chicken
**Preparation Time: 15 Minutes**
**Cooking Time:** 25 Minutes
**Servings: 3**

**Ingredients:**
2 medium mangoes, peeled and sliced
10ounce coconut almond milk
4 teaspoons vegetable oil
4 teaspoons spicy curry paste
14ounce chicken breast halves, skinless and boneless, cut in cubes
4 medium shallots
1 large English cucumber, sliced and seeded

**Directions:**
Slice half of the mangoes and add the halves to a bowl.
Add mangoes and coconut almond milk to a blender and blend until you have a smooth puree.
Keep the mixture on the side.
Take a largesized pot and place it over medium heat, add oil and allow the oil to heat up.
Add curry paste and cook for 1 minute until you have a nice fragrance, add shallots and chicken to the pot and cook for 5 minutes.
Pour mango puree in to the mix and allow it to heat up.
Serve the cooked chicken with mango puree and cucumbers.
Enjoy!

**Nutrition:**
Calories: 398
Fat: 20g
Carbohydrates: 32g
Protein: 26g

## 147. Chicken and Cabbage Platter

**Preparation Time: 15 Minutes**
**Cooking Time:** 25 Minutes
**Servings: 3**
**Ingredients:**
1/2 cup sliced onion
1 tablespoon sesame garlicflavored oil
2 cups shredded BokChoy
1/2 cups fresh bean sprouts
1 1/2 stalks celery, chopped
1 1/2 teaspoons minced garlic
1/2 teaspoon stevia
1/2 cup chicken broth
1 tablespoon coconut aminos
1/2 tablespoon freshly minced ginger
1/2 teaspoon arrowroot
2 boneless chicken breasts, cooked and sliced thinly

**Directions:**
Shred the cabbage with a knife.
Slice onion and add to your platter alongside the rotisserie chicken.
Add a dollop of mayonnaise on top and drizzle olive oil over the cabbage.
Season with sunflower seeds and pepper according to your taste.
Enjoy!

**Nutrition:**
Calories: 368
Fat: 18g
Net Carbohydrates: 8g
Protein: 42g
Fiber: 3g
Carbohydrates: 11g

## 148. Hearty Chicken Liver Stew

**Preparation Time: 15 Minutes**
**Cooking Time:** 25 Minutes
**Servings: 3**
**Ingredients:**
10 ounces chicken livers
1ounce onion, chopped
2 ounces sour cream
1 tablespoon olive oil
Sunflower seeds to taste

**Directions:**
Take a pan and place it over medium heat.
Add oil and let it heat up.
Add onions and fry until just browned.
Add livers and season with sunflower seeds.
Cook until livers are half cooked.

Transfer the mix to a stew pot.
Add sour cream and cook for 20 minutes.

Serve and enjoy!
**Nutrition:**
Calories: 146
Fat: 9g
Carbohydrates: 2g
Protein: 15g

## 149. Chicken Quesadilla
**Preparation Time: 15 Minutes**
**Cooking Time:** 25 Minutes
**Servings: 3**
**Ingredients:**
1/4 cup ranch dressing
1/2 cup cheddar cheese, shredded
20 slices bacon, centercut
2 cups Steamed chicken, sliced
**Directions:**
Reheat your oven to 400 degrees F.
Line baking sheet using parchment paper.
Weave bacon into two rectangles and bake for 30 minutes.
Lay Steamed chicken over bacon square, drizzling ranch dressing on top.
Sprinkle cheddar cheese and top with another bacon square.
Bake for 5 minutes more.
Slice and serve.
Enjoy!
**Nutrition:**
Calories: 619
Fat: 35g
Carbohydrates: 2g
Protein: 79g

## 150. Mustard Chicken
**Preparation Time: 15 Minutes**
**Cooking Time:** 25 Minutes
**Servings: 3**
**Ingredients:**
2 chicken breasts
1/4 cup chicken broth
2 tablespoons mustard
1 1/2 tablespoons olive oil
1/2 teaspoon paprika

1/2 teaspoon chili powder
1/2 teaspoon garlic powder
**Directions:**
Take a small bowl and mix mustard, olive oil, paprika, chicken broth, garlic powder, chicken broth, and chili.
Add chicken breast and marinate for 30 minutes.
Take a lined baking sheet and arrange the chicken.
Bake for 35 minutes at 375 degrees F.
Serve and enjoy!
**Nutrition:**
Calories: 531
Fat: 23g
Carbohydrates: 10g
Protein: 64g

## 151. Chicken and Carrot Stew
**Preparation Time: 15 Minutes**
**Cooking Time:** 25 Minutes
**Servings: 3**
**Ingredients:**
4 boneless chicken breast, cubed
3 cups of carrots, peeled and cubed
1 cup onion, chopped
1 cup tomatoes, chopped
1 teaspoon of dried thyme
2 cups of chicken broth
2 garlic cloves, minced
Sunflower seeds and pepper as needed
**Directions:**
Add all of the listed ingredients to a Slow Cooker.
Stir and close the lid.
Cook for 6 hours.
Serve hot and enjoy!
**Nutrition:**
Calories: 182
Fat: 3g
Carbohydrates: 10g
Protein: 39g

## 152. The Delish Turkey Wrap
**Preparation Time: 15 Minutes**
**Cooking Time:** 25 Minutes
**Servings: 3**
**Ingredients:**
1 1/4 pounds ground turkey, lean
4 green onions, minced
1 tablespoon olive oil
1 garlic clove, minced
2 teaspoons chili paste
8ounce water chestnut, diced
3 tablespoons hoisin sauce
2 tablespoon coconut aminos
1 tablespoon rice vinegar
12 almond butter lettuce leaves
1/8 teaspoon sunflower seeds
**Directions:**
Take a pan and place it over medium heat, add turkey and garlic to the pan.
Heat for 6 minutes until cooked.
Take a bowl and transfer turkey to the bowl.
Add onions and water chestnuts.
Stir in hoisin sauce, coconut aminos, vinegar and chili paste.
Toss well and transfer mix to lettuce leaves.
Serve and enjoy!
**Nutrition:**
Calories: 162
Fat: 4g
Net Carbohydrates: 7g
Protein: 23g

## 153. Almond butternut Chicken
**Preparation Time: 15 Minutes**
**Cooking Time:** 25 Minutes
**Servings: 3**
**Ingredients:**
1/2 pound Nitrate free bacon
6 chicken thighs, boneless and skinless
23 cups almond butternut squash, cubed
Extra virgin olive oil
Fresh chopped sage
Sunflower seeds and pepper as needed
**Directions:**
Prepare your oven by preheating it to 425 degrees F.
Take a large skillet and place it over mediumhigh heat, add bacon and fry until crispy.
Take a slice of bacon and place it on the side, crumble the bacon.
Add cubed almond butternut squash in the bacon grease and sauté, season with sunflower seeds and pepper.
Once the squash is tender, remove skillet and transfer to a plate.
Add coconut oil to the skillet and add chicken thighs, cook for 10 minutes.
Season with sunflower seeds and pepper.
Remove skillet from stove and transfer to oven.
Bake for 1215 minutes, top with the crumbled bacon and sage.
Enjoy!
**Nutrition:**
Calories: 323
Fat: 19g
Carbohydrates: 8g
Protein: 12g

## 154. Duck with Cucumber and Carrots
**Preparation Time: 15 Minutes**
**Cooking Time:** 25 Minutes
**Servings: 3**
**Ingredients:**
1 duck, cut up into medium pieces
1 chopped cucumber, chopped
1 tablespoon low sodium vegetable stock
2 carrots, chopped
2 cups of water

Black pepper as needed
1inch ginger piece, grated
**Directions:**
Add duck pieces to your Instant Pot.
Add cucumber, stock, carrots, water, ginger, pepper and stir.
Lock up the lid and cook on LOW pressure for 40 minutes.
Release the pressure naturally.
Serve and enjoy!
**Nutrition:**
Calories: 206
Fats: 7g
Carbs: 28g
Protein: 16g

### 155. Anchovy Parmesan Pasta

**Preparation Time: 15 Minutes**
**Cooking Time:** 25 Minutes
**Servings: 3**
**Ingredients:**
4 anchovy fillets, packed in olive oil
1/2 pound broccoli, cut into 1inch florets
2 cloves garlic, sliced
1pound wholewheat penne
2 tablespoons olive oil
1/4 cup Parmesan cheese, grated
Salt and black pepper, to taste
Red pepper flakes, to taste
**Directions:**
Cook pasta as directed over pack; drain and set aside. Take a medium saucepan or skillet, add oil. Heat over medium heat.
Add anchovies, broccoli, and garlic, and stircook until veggies turn tender for 45 minutes. Take off heat; mix in the pasta. Serve warm with Parmesan cheese, red pepper flakes, salt, and black pepper sprinkled on top.
**Nutrition:**
Calories 328
Fat 8g

Carbohydrates 35g
Protein 7g

### 156. GarlicShrimp Pasta
**Preparation Time: 15 Minutes**
**Cooking Time:** 25 Minutes
**Servings: 3**
**Ingredients:**
1pound shrimp, peeled and deveined
3 garlic cloves, minced
1 onion, finely chopped
1 package whole wheat or bean pasta of your choice
4 tablespoons olive oil
Salt and black pepper, to taste
1/4 cup basil, cut into strips
3/4 cup chicken broth, lowsodium
**Directions:**
Cook pasta as directed over pack; rinse and set aside. Get medium saucepan, add oil then warm up over medium heat. Add onion, garlic and stircook until become translucent and fragrant for 3 minutes.
Add shrimp, black pepper (ground) and salt; stircook for 3 minutes until shrimps are opaque. Add broth and simmer for 23 more minutes. Add pasta in serving plates; add shrimp mixture over; serve warm with basil on top.
**Nutrition:**
Calories 605
Fat 17g
Carbohydrates 53g
Protein 19g

### 157. Simple Pesto Pasta
**Preparation Time: 15 Minutes**
**Cooking Time:** 25 Minutes
**Servings: 3**
**Ingredients:**
1 lb. spaghetti
4 cups fresh basil leaves, stems removed

---

3 cloves garlic
1 tsp. salt
1/2 tsp. freshly ground black pepper
1/4 cup lemon juice
1/2 cup pine nuts, toasted
1/2 cup grated Parmesan cheese
1 cup extravirgin olive oil

**Directions:**

Bring a large pot of salted water to a boil. Add the spaghetti to the pot and cook for 8 minutes.

Put basil, garlic, salt, pepper, lemon juice, pine nuts, and Parmesan cheese in a food processor bowl with chopping blade and purée.

While the processor is running, slowly drizzle the olive oil through the top opening. Process until all the olive oil has been added.

Reserve 1/2 cup of the pasta water. Drain the pasta and put it into a bowl. Immediately add the pesto and pasta water to the pasta and toss everything together. Serve warm.

**Nutrition:**
Calories: 280
Fat: 8g
Protein: 8g
Carbs: 46g
Fiber: 9g
Sodium: 200mg

## 158. Meaty Baked Penne

**Preparation Time: 15 Minutes**
**Cooking Time:** 25 Minutes
**Servings: 3**
**Ingredients:**
1 lb. penne pasta
1 lb. ground beef
1 tsp. salt
1 (25oz.) jar marinara sauce
1 (1lb.) bag baby spinach, washed
3 cups shredded mozzarella cheese, divided

**Directions:**

Bring a large pot of salted water to a boil, add the penne, and cook for 7 minutes. Reserve 2 cups of e pasta water and drain the pasta.

Preheat the oven to 350°F.

In a large saucepan over medium heat, cook the ground beef and salt. Brown the ground beef for about 5 minutes.

Stir in marinara sauce, and 2 cups of pasta water. Let simmer for 5 minutes.

Add a handful of spinach at a time into the sauce, and cook for another 3 minutes.

To assemble, in a 9by13inch baking dish, add the pasta and pour the pasta sauce over it. Stir in 11/2 cups of the mozzarella cheese. Cover the dish with foil and bake for 20 minutes.

After 20 minutes, remove the foil, top with the rest of the mozzarella, and bake for another 10 minutes. Serve warm.

**Nutrition:**
Calories 285
Fat 9.1 g
Carbohydrates 45.7 g
Sugar 1.2 g
Protein 6 g
Cholesterol 0 mg

## 159. Mediterranean Pasta with Tomato Sauce and Vegetables

**Preparation Time: 15 Minutes**
**Cooking Time:** 25 Minutes
**Servings: 3**
**Ingredients:**
8 oz. linguine or spaghetti, cooked
1 tsp. garlic powder
1 (28 oz.) can whole peeled tomatoes, drained and sliced
1 tbsp. olive oil
1 (8 oz.) can tomato sauce
1/2 tsp. Italian seasoning
8 oz. mushrooms, sliced

~ 118 ~

8 oz. yellow squash, sliced
8 oz. zucchini, sliced
1/2 tsp. sugar
1/2 cup grated Parmesan cheese

**Directions:**

In a medium saucepan, mix tomato sauce, tomatoes, sugar, Italian seasoning, and garlic powder. Bring to boil on medium heat. Reduce heat to low. Cover and simmer for 20 minutes. In a large skillet, heat olive oil on mediumhigh heat.

Add squash, mushrooms, and zucchini. Cook, stirring, for 4 minutes or until tendercrisp.

Stir vegetables into the tomato sauce.

Place pasta in a serving bowl.

Spoon vegetable mixture over pasta and toss to coat.

Top with grated Parmesan cheese.

**Nutrition:**

Calories : 212

Carbs: 30.6g

Protein: 15.9g

Fat: 3.0g

## 160. Very Vegan Patras Pasta

**Preparation Time: 15 Minutes**

**Cooking Time:** 25 Minutes

**Servings: 3**

**Ingredients:**

4quarts salted water

10oz. glutenfree and wholegrain pasta

5cloves garlic, minced

1cup hummus

Salt and pepper

1/3cup water

1/2cup walnuts

1/2cup olives

2tbsp dried cranberries (optional)

**Directions:**

Bring the salted water to a boil for cooking the pasta.

In the meantime, prepare for the hummus sauce. Combine the garlic, hummus, salt, and pepper with water in a mixing bowl. Add the walnuts,

olive, and dried cranberries, if desired. Set aside.

Add the pasta in the boiling water. Cook the pasta following the manufacturer's specifications until attaining an al dente texture. Drain the pasta.

Transfer the pasta to a large serving bowl and combine with the sauce.

**Nutrition:**

Calories : 207.4

Carbs: 31g

Protein: 5.1g

Fat: 7g

## 161. Cheesy Spaghetti with Pine Nuts

**Preparation Time: 15 Minutes**

**Cooking Time:** 25 Minutes

**Servings: 3**

**Ingredients:**

8 oz. spaghetti

4 tbsp. (1/2 stick) unsalted butter

1 tsp. freshly ground black pepper

1/2 cup pine nuts

1 cup fresh grated Parmesan cheese, divided

**Directions:**

Bring a large pot of salted water to a boil. Add the pasta and cook for 8 minutes.

In a large saucepan over medium heat, combine the butter, black pepper, and pine nuts. Cook for 2 to 3 minutes or until the pine nuts are lightly toasted.

Reserve 1/2 cup of the pasta water. Drain the pasta and put it into the pan with the pine nuts.

Add 3/4 cup of Parmesan cheese and the reserved pasta water to the pasta and toss everything together to evenly coat the pasta.

To serve, put the pasta in a serving dish and top with the remaining 1/4 cup of Parmesan cheese.

**Nutrition:**
Calories: 249 Carbs: 31.0g
Protein: 8.0g Fat: 10.0g

## 162. Creamy Garlic Parmesan Chicken Pasta

**Preparation Time: 15 Minutes**
**Cooking Time:** 25 Minutes
**Servings: 3**
**Ingredients:**
2 boneless, skinless chicken breasts
3 tbsp. extra-virgin olive oil
11/2 tsp. salt
1 large onion, thinly sliced
3 tbsp. garlic, minced
1 lb. fettuccine pasta
1 cup heavy (whipping) cream
3/4 cup freshly grated Parmesan cheese, divided
1/2 tsp. freshly ground black pepper
**Directions:**
Bring a large pot of salted water to a simmer.
Cut the chicken into thin strips.
In a large skillet over medium heat, cook the olive oil and chicken for 3 minutes.
Next add the salt, onion, and garlic to the pan with the chicken. Cook for 7 minutes.
Bring the pot of salted water to a boil and add the pasta, then let it cook for 7 minutes.
While the pasta is cooking, add the cream, 1/2 cup of Parmesan cheese, and black pepper to the chicken; simmer for 3 minutes.
Reserve 1/2 cup of the pasta water. Drain the pasta and add it to the chicken cream sauce.
Add the reserved pasta water to the pasta and toss together. Let simmer for 2 minutes. Top with the remaining 1/4 cup Parmesan cheese and serve warm.
**Nutrition:**

Calories: 357 Carbs: 39.0g
Protein: 16.7g
Fat: 15.9g

## 163. P Chicken Spinach and Artichoke Stuffed Spaghetti Squash

**Preparation Time: 15 Minutes**
**Cooking Time:** 25 Minutes
**Servings: 3**
**Ingredients:**
4 oz reducedfat cream cheese, cubed and softened
1/4 tsp ground pepper
3 tbsp water
1/4 tsp salt
Crushed red peppers
3 lb spaghetti squash, halved lengthwise and seeded
1/2 cup shredded parmesan cheese
5 oz pack baby spinach
10 oz pack artichoke hearts, chopped
Diced fresh basil
**Directions:**
On a microwaveable dish, place your squash halves with the cut side facing up. Add 2 tbsp of water to the squash. Set the microwave to high and cook without covering the dish for about 15 minutes. You can also place the squash on a prepared baking sheet (rimmed) and bake at 400 degrees F for 40 minutes.
Set your stove to medium heat and place a large skillet containing 1 tbsp of water on it. Add spinach into the pan and stir while it cooks for about 5 minutes, or until the vegetable wilts. Drain the spinach and place in a bowl.
Place the rack in the upper third region of your oven, then preheat your broiler.
Using a fork, scrape squash from each shell half, and place them in a bowl. Add artichoke hearts, pepper, salt,

cream cheese, and 1/4 cup parmesan into the bowl of squash. Mix well. Place squash shells on a baking sheet and add the squash mixture into the shells. Add the remaining parmesan on top and broil for 3 minutes.

Garnish with red pepper and basil and serve.

**Nutrition:**
Calories: 324.4
 Protein: 22g
Carbs: 33g
Fat: 11.6g

# 164. Angel Hair with AsparagusKale Pesto
**Preparation Time: 15 Minutes**
**Cooking Time:** 25 Minutes
**Servings: 3**
**Ingredients:**
3/4pound asparagus, woody ends removed, and coarsely chopped
1/4pound kale, thoroughly washed
1/2 cup grated Asiago cheese
1/4 cup fresh basil
1/4 cup extravirgin olive oil
Juice of 1 lemon
Sea salt
Freshly ground black pepper
1pound angel hair pasta
Zest of 1 lemon
**Directions:**
In a food processor, pulse the asparagus and kale until very finely chopped.
Add the Asiago cheese, basil, olive oil, and lemon juice and pulse to form a smooth pesto.
Season with sea salt and pepper and set aside.
Cook the pasta al dente according to the package directions. Drain and transfer to a large bowl.
Add the pesto, tossing well to coat
Sprinkle with lemon zest and serve.

Cooking tip: You can make the asparagus pesto up to 3 days ahead. Keep it refrigerated until you need it.

**Nutrition:**
Calories: 376
Carbs: 50.8g
Protein: 17.8g
Fat: 11.6g

# 165. Spicy Pasta Puttanesca
**Preparation Time: 15 Minutes**
**Cooking Time:** 25 Minutes
**Servings: 3**
**Ingredients:**
2 teaspoons extravirgin olive oil
1/2 sweet onion, finely chopped
2 teaspoons minced garlic
1 (28ounce) can sodiumfree diced tomatoes
1/2 cup chopped anchovies
2 teaspoons chopped fresh oregano
2 teaspoons chopped fresh basil
1/2 teaspoon red pepper flakes
1/2 cup quartered Kalamata olives
1/4 cup sodiumfree chicken broth
1 tablespoon capers, drained and rinsed
Juice of 1 lemon
4 cups cooked wholegrain penne
**Directions:**
In a large saucepan over medium heat, heat the olive oil.
Add the onion and garlic, and sauté for about 3 minutes until softened.
Stir in the tomatoes, anchovies, oregano, basil, and red pepper flakes. Bring the sauce to a boil and reduce the heat to low. Simmer for 15 minutes, stirring occasionally.
Stir in the olives, chicken broth, capers, and lemon juice.
Cook the pasta according to the

package directions and serve topped with the sauce.

Ingredient tip: Do not mistake sardines for anchovies, although they are both small, silvery fish sold in cans. Anchovies are usually salted in brine and matured to create a distinctive, rich taste.

**Nutrition:**
Calories: 274.7
Carbs: 30.9g
Protein: 14.6g
Fat: 10.3g

## 166. Roasted Vegetarian Lasagna

**Preparation Time: 15 Minutes**
**Cooking Time:** 25 Minutes
**Servings: 3**
Ingredients:
1 eggplant, thickly sliced
2 zucchini, sliced lengthwise
1 yellow squash, sliced lengthwise
1 sweet onion, thickly sliced
2 tablespoons extravirgin olive oil
1 (28ounce) can sodiumfree diced tomatoes
1 cup quartered, canned, waterpacked artichoke hearts, drained
2 teaspoons minced garlic
2 teaspoons chopped fresh basil
2 teaspoons chopped fresh oregano
Pinch red pepper flakes
12 noboil wholegrain lasagna noodles
3/4 cup grated Asiago cheese
**Directions:**
Preheat the oven to 400°F.
Line a baking sheet with aluminum foil and set aside.
In a large bowl, toss together the eggplant, zucchini, yellow squash, onion, and olive oil to coat.
Arrange the vegetables on the prepared sheet and roast for about 20 minutes, or until tender and lightly caramelized.

Chop the roasted vegetables well and transfer them to a large bowl.

Stir in the tomatoes, artichoke hearts, garlic, basil, oregano, and red pepper flakes

Spoon onequarter of the vegetable mixture into the bottom of a deep 9by13inch baking dish.

Arrange 4 lasagna noodles over the sauce.

Repeat, alternating sauce and noodles, ending with sauce.

Sprinkle the Asiago cheese evenly over the top. Bake for about 30 minutes until bubbly and hot.

Remove from the oven and cool for 15 minutes before serving.

Substitution tip: If having a vegetarian meal is not a requirement, lean ground beef (92%) or ground chicken can be added to the roasted vegetable sauce for a more robust meal. Brown the ground meat in a skillet and add it to the finished sauce before assembling the lasagna.

**Nutrition:**
Calories: 456.6
Carbs: 77.3g
Protein: 16.6g
Fat: 9g

## 167. Cauliflower Tabbouleh

**Preparation Time: 15 Minutes**
**Cooking Time:** 25 Minutes
**Servings: 3**
**Ingredients:**
6 tablespoons extra virgin olive oil, divided
4 cups Riced Cauliflower
3 garlic cloves, finely minced
11/2 teaspoons salt
1/2 teaspoon freshly ground black pepper
1/2 large cucumber, peeled, seeded, and chopped

1/2 cup chopped mint leaves
1/2 cup chopped Italian parsley
1/2 cup chopped pitted Kalamata olives
2 tablespoons minced red onion
Juice of 1 lemon (about 2 tablespoons)
2 cups baby arugula or spinach leaves
2 medium avocados, peeled, pitted, and diced
1 cup quartered cherry tomatoes
**Directions:**
In a large skillet, heat 2 tablespoons of olive oil over medium high heat. Add the riced cauliflower, garlic, salt, and pepper and sauté until just tender but not mushy, 3 to 4 minutes. Remove from the heat and place in a large bowl. salt and Add the cucumber, mint, parsley, olives, red onion, lemon juice, and remaining 4 tablespoons olive oil and toss well. Place in the refrigerator, uncovered, and refrigerate for at least 30 minutes, or up to 2 hours.
Before serving, add the arugula, avocado, and tomatoes and toss to combine well. Season to taste with pepper and serve cold or at room temperature.
**Nutrition:**
Calories: 235
Total Fat: 21g,
Total Carbs: 12g,
Net Carbs: 6g,
Fiber: 6g
Protein: 4g
Sodium: 623mg

## 168. Garlicky Broccoli Rabe with Artichokes
**Preparation Time:** 15 Minutes
**Cooking Time:** 25 Minutes
**Servings:** 3
**Ingredients:**
2 pounds fresh broccoli rabe
1/2 cup extravirgin olive oil, divided

3 garlic cloves, finely minced
1 teaspoon salt
1 teaspoon red pepper flakes
1 (13.75ounce) can artichoke hearts, drained and quartered
1 tablespoon water
2 tablespoons red wine vinegar
Freshly ground black pepper
**Directions:**
Trim away any thick lower stems and yellow leaves from the broccoli rabe and discard. Cut into individual florets with a couple inches of thin stem attached.
2.In a large skillet, heat 1/4 cup olive oil over mediumhigh heat. Add the trimmed broccoli, garlic, salt, and red pepper flakes and sauté for 5 minutes, until the broccoli begins to soften. Add the artichoke hearts and sauté for another 2 minutes.
3.Add the water and reduce the heat to low. Cover and simmer until the broccoli stems are tender, 3 to 5 minutes.
4.In a small bowl, whisk together remaining 1/4 cup olive oil and the vinegar. Drizzle over the broccoli and artichokes. Season with ground black pepper, if desired.
**Nutrition:**
Calories: 385
Total Fat: 35g
Total Carbs: 18g
Net Carbs: 8g
Fiber: 10g
Protein: 11g
Sodium: 918g

## 169. Roasted Eggplant with Mint and Harissa
**Preparation Time:** 15 Minutes
**Cooking Time:** 25 Minutes
**Servings:** 3
**Ingredients:**

2 medium eggplants, cut into 1/2inch cubes

4 tablespoons extravirgin olive oil

1 teaspoon salt

1/4 teaspoon freshly ground black pepper

1 cup chopped fresh mint

1/4 cup Harissa Oil or storebought harissa

1/4 cup chopped scallions, green part only

**Directions:**

Preheat the oven to 425°F. Line a baking sheet with parchment paper.

2.In a large bowl, place the eggplant, olive oil, salt, and pepper and toss to coat well.

3.Place the eggplant on the prepared baking sheet, reserving the bowl, and roast for 15 minutes. Remove from the oven and toss the eggplant pieces to flip. Return to the oven and roast until golden and cooked through, another 15 to 20 minutes.

4.When the eggplant is cooked, remove from the oven and return to the large bowl. Add the mint, harissa, and scallions and toss to combine. Serve warm or cover and refrigerate for up to 2 days.

**Nutrition:**

Calories: 300

Total Fat: 28g

Total Carbs: 15g

Net Carbs: 7g

Fiber: 8g

## 170. Shakshuka

**Preparation Time: 15 Minutes**

**Cooking Time:** 25 Minutes

**Servings: 3**

**Ingredients:**

1/2 cup plus 2 tablespoons extravirgin olive oil, divided

1/2 small yellow onion, finely diced

1 red bell pepper, finely diced

1 (14ounce) can crushed tomatoes, with juices

6 ounces frozen spinach, thawed and drained of excess liquid (about 11/2 cups)

2 garlic cloves, finely minced

1 teaspoon smoked paprika

1 to 2 teaspoons red pepper flakes (optional)

1 tablespoon roughly chopped capers

6 large eggs

1/4 teaspoon freshly ground black pepper

3/4 cup crumbled feta or goat cheese

1/4 cup chopped fresh flatleaf parsley or cilantro

**Directions:**

Heat broiler on low setting.

2.In a medium, deep ovensafe skillet, heat 2 tablespoons olive oil over mediumhigh heat. Add the onion and bell pepper and sauté until softened, 5 to 8 minutes.

3.Add the crushed tomatoes and their juices, 1/2 cup olive oil, spinach, garlic, paprika, red pepper flakes (if using), and capers, stirring to combine. Bring to a boil, then reduce the heat to low, cover, and simmer for 5 minutes.

4.Uncover the pan and gently crack each egg into the simmering sauce, allowing the egg to create a crater in the sauce and being careful to not let eggs touch. Add the pepper, then cover and cook, poaching the eggs until the yolks are just set, eight to 10 minutes. Eight minutes will yield softer yolks, while a longer cooking time will yield firmer yolks.

5.Uncover the pan and spread the crumbled cheese over top of the eggs and sauce. Transfer to the oven and broil under low heat until the cheese is just slightly browned and bubbly, 3 to 5 minutes. Drizzle with the remaining 2 tablespoons olive oil, top with chopped parsley, and serve warm.

Prep Tip: For an even quicker preparation, substitute 1 jar lowsugar marinara sauce (less than 6 grams) for the onion, bell pepper, crushed tomatoes, and garlic. Skip steps 2 and 3, season the marinara sauce with paprika and red pepper flakes, and bring to a simmer before cracking in the eggs.

**Nutrition:**
Calories: 476,
Total Fat: 40g,
 Total Carbs: 12g,
Net Carbs: 7g,
Fiber: 5g,
Protein: 17g;
Sodium: 287mg
Macros: Fat: 76%, Carbs: 10%, Protein: 14%

## 171. Crustless Spanakopita
**Preparation Time: 15 Minutes**
**Cooking Time:** 25 Minutes
**Servings: 3**
**Ingredients:**
12 tablespoons extravirgin olive oil, divided
1 small yellow onion, diced
1 (32ounce) bag frozen chopped spinach, thawed, fully drained, and patted dry (about 4 cups)
4 garlic cloves, minced
1/2 teaspoon salt
1/2 teaspoon freshly ground black pepper
1 cup wholemilk ricotta cheese
4 large eggs
3/4 cup crumbled traditional feta cheese
1/4 cup pine nuts
**Directions:**
Preheat the oven to 375°F.

In a large skillet, heat 4 tablespoons olive oil over mediumhigh heat. Add the onion and sauté until softened, 6 to 8 minutes.

Add the spinach, garlic, salt, and pepper and sauté another 5 minutes. Remove from the heat and allow to cool slightly.

In a medium bowl, whisk together the ricotta and eggs. Add to the cooled spinach and stir to combine.

Pour 4 tablespoons olive oil in the bottom of a 9by13inch glass baking dish and swirl to coat the bottom and sides. Add the spinachricotta mixture and spread into an even layer.

Bake for 20 minutes or until the mixture begins to set. Remove from the oven and crumble the feta evenly across the top of the spinach. Add the pine nuts and drizzle with the remaining 4 tablespoons olive oil. Return to the oven and bake for an additional 15 to 20 minutes, or until the spinach is fully set and the top is starting to turn golden brown. Allow to cool slightly before cutting to serve.

**Nutrition:**
Calories: 484,
 Total Fat: 43g,
Total Carbs: 10g,
 Net Carbs: 5g,
Fiber: 5g,
Protein: 18g;
Sodium: 438mg
Macros: Fat: 79%, Carbs: 8%, Protein: 13%

## 172. Zucchini Lasagna
**Preparation Time: 15 Minutes**
**Cooking Time:** 25 Minutes
**Servings: 3**
**Ingredients:**
1/2 cup extravirgin olive oil, divided
4 to 5 medium zucchini squash

1 teaspoon salt

8 ounces frozen spinach, thawed and well drained (about 1 cup)

2 cups wholemilk ricotta cheese

1/4 cup chopped fresh basil or 2 teaspoons dried basil

1 teaspoon garlic powder

1/2 teaspoon freshly ground black pepper

2 cups shredded fresh wholemilk mozzarella cheese

13/4 cups shredded Parmesan cheese

1/2 (24ounce) jar lowsugar marinara sauce (less than 5 grams sugar)

**Directions:**

.Preheat the oven to 425°F.

2.Line two baking sheets with parchment paper or aluminum foil and drizzle each with 2 tablespoons olive oil, spreading evenly.

3.Slice the zucchini lengthwise into 1/4inchthick long slices and place on the prepared baking sheet in a single layer. Sprinkle with 1/2 teaspoon salt per sheet. Bake until softened, but not mushy, 15 to 18 minutes. Remove from the oven and allow to cool slightly before assembling the lasagna.

4.Reduce the oven temperature to 375°F.

5.While the zucchini cooks, prep the filling. In a large bowl, combine the spinach, ricotta, basil, garlic powder, and pepper. In a small bowl, mix together the mozzarella and Parmesan cheeses. In a medium bowl, combine the marinara sauce and remaining 1/4 cup olive oil and stir to fully incorporate the oil into sauce.

6.To assemble the lasagna, spoon a third of the marinara sauce mixture into the bottom of a 9by13inch glass baking dish and spread evenly. Place 1 layer of softened zucchini slices to fully cover the sauce, then add a third of the ricottaspinach mixture and spread evenly on top of the zucchini. Sprinkle a third of the mozzarellaParmesan mixture on top of the ricotta. Repeat with 2 more cycles of these layers: marinara, zucchini, ricottaspinach, then cheese blend.

7.Bake until the cheese is bubbly and melted, 30 to 35 minutes. Turn the broiler to low and broil until the top is golden brown, about 5 minutes. Remove from the oven and allow to cool slightly before slicing.

**Nutrition:**

Calories: 521, Total Fat: 41g,

Total Carbs: 13g, Net Carbs: 10g,

Fiber: 3g,

Protein: 25g; Sodium: 712mg

Macros: Fat: 71%, Carbs: 10%, Protein: 19%

## 173. Moroccan Vegetable Tagine

**Preparation Time: 15 Minutes**

**Cooking Time:** 25 Minutes

**Servings: 3**

**Ingredients:**

1/2 cup extravirgin olive oil

2 medium yellow onions, sliced

6 celery stalks, sliced into 1/4inch crescents

6 garlic cloves, minced

1 teaspoon ground cumin

1 teaspoon ginger powder

1 teaspoon salt

1/2 teaspoon paprika

1/2 teaspoon ground cinnamon

1/4 teaspoon freshly ground black pepper

2 cups vegetable stock

1 medium eggplant, cut into 1inch cubes

2 medium zucchini, cut into 1/2inchthick semicircles

2 cups cauliflower florets
1 (13.75ounce) can artichoke hearts, drained and quartered
1 cup halved and pitted green olives
1/2 cup chopped fresh flatleaf parsley, for garnish
1/2 cup chopped fresh cilantro leaves, for garnish
Greek yogurt, for garnish (optional)
**Directions:**
.In a large, thick soup pot or Dutch oven, heat the olive oil over medium high heat. Add the onion and celery and sauté until softened, 6 to 8 minutes. Add the garlic, cumin, ginger, salt, paprika, cinnamon, and pepper and sauté for another 2 minutes.
2.Add the stock and bring to a boil. Reduce the heat to low and add the eggplant, zucchini, and cauliflower. Simmer on low heat, covered, until the vegetables are tender, 30 to 35 minutes. Add the artichoke hearts and olives, cover, and simmer for another 15 minutes.
3.Serve garnished with parsley, cilantro, and Greek yogurt (if using).
Substitution Tip: You can replace the spice combination used in this recipe with garam masala, an Indian spice blend found in many grocery stores.
**Nutrition:**
Calories: 309, Total Fat: 21g,
Total Carbs: 24g, Net Carbs: 15g,
Fiber: 9g, Protein: 6g;
 Sodium: 1167mg
Macros: Fat: 61%, Carbs: 12%, Protein: 27%

## 174. Citrus Asparagus with Pistachios
**Preparation Time: 15 Minutes**
**Cooking Time:** 25 Minutes
**Servings: 3**
**Ingredients:**

5 tablespoons extra virgin olive oil, divided
Zest and juice of 2 clementine's or 1 orange (about 1/4 cup juice and 1 tablespoon zest)
Zest and juice of 1 lemon
1 tablespoon red wine vinegar
1 teaspoon salt, divided
1/4 teaspoon freshly ground black pepper
1/2 cup shelled pistachios
1 pound fresh asparagus
 1 tablespoon water
**Directions:**
.In a small bowl, whisk together 4 tablespoons olive oil, the clementine and lemon juices and zests, vinegar, 1/2 teaspoon salt, and pepper. Set aside.
2.In a medium dry skillet, toast the pistachios over medium high heat until lightly browned, 2 to 3 minutes, being careful not to let them burn. Transfer to a cutting board and coarsely chop. Set aside.
3.Trim the rough ends off the asparagus, usually the last 1 to 2 inches of each spear. In a skillet, heat the remaining 1 tablespoon olive oil over medium high heat. Add the asparagus and sauté for 2 to 3 minutes. Sprinkle with the remaining 1/2 teaspoon salt and add the water. Reduce the heat to medium low, cover, and cook until tender, another 2 to 4 minutes, depending on the thickness of the spears.
4.Transfer the cooked asparagus to a serving dish. Add the pistachios to the dressing and whisk to combine. Pour the dressing over the warm asparagus and toss to coat.
**Nutrition:**
Calories: 284, Total Fat: 24g

Total Carbs: 11g Net Carbs: 7g,
Fiber: 4g Protein: 6g
 Sodium: 594mg Macros: Fat: 76%,
Carbs: 15%, Protein: 9%

Fiber: 2g, Protein: 7g;
Sodium: 325mg
Macros: Fat: 79%, Carbs: 11%,
Protein: 10%

## 175. Herbed Ricotta–Stuffed Mushrooms

**Preparation Time:** 15 Minutes
**Cooking Time:** 25 Minutes
**Servings: 3**
**Ingredients:**
6 tablespoons extra virgin olive oil, divided
4 portobello mushroom caps, cleaned and gills removed
1 cup whole milk ricotta cheese
1/3 cup chopped fresh herbs (such as basil, parsley, rosemary, oregano, or thyme)
2 garlic cloves, finely minced
1/2 teaspoon salt
1/4 teaspoon freshly ground black pepper
**Directions:**
Preheat the oven to 400°F.
2.Line a baking sheet with parchment or foil and drizzle with 2 tablespoons olive oil, spreading evenly. Place the mushroom caps on the baking sheet, gill side up.
3.In a medium bowl, mix together the ricotta, herbs, 2 tablespoons olive oil, garlic, salt, and pepper. Stuff each mushroom cap with one quarter of the cheese mixture, pressing down if needed. Drizzle with remaining 2 tablespoons olive oil and bake until golden brown and the mushrooms are soft, 30 to 35 minutes, depending on the size of the mushrooms.
**Nutrition:**
Calories: 285,
Total Fat: 25g,
Total Carbs: 8g,
Net Carbs: 6g,

## 176. Braised Greens with Olives and Walnuts

**Preparation Time:** 15 Minutes
**Cooking Time:** 25 Minutes
**Servings: 3**
**Ingredients:**
8 cups fresh greens (such as kale, mustard greens, spinach, or chard)
2 to 4 garlic cloves, finely minced
1/2 cup roughly chopped pitted green or black olives
1/2 cup roughly chopped shelled walnuts - 1/4 cup extra virgin olive oil
2 tablespoons red wine vinegar
1 to 2 teaspoons freshly chopped herbs such as oregano, basil, rosemary, or thyme
**Directions:**
Remove the tough stems from the greens and chop into bitesize pieces. Place in a large rimmed skillet or pot.
2.Turn the heat to high and add the minced garlic and enough water to just cover the greens. Bring to a boil, reduce the heat to low, and simmer until the greens are wilted and tender and most of the liquid has evaporated, adding more if the greens start to burn. For more tender greens such as spinach, this may only take 5 minutes, while tougher greens such as chard may need up to 20 minutes. Once cooked, remove from the heat and add the chopped olives and walnuts.
3.In a small bowl, whisk together olive oil, vinegar, and herbs. Drizzle over the cooked greens and toss to coat. Serve warm.
**Nutrition:**
Calories: 280, Total Fat: 20g,

Total Carbs: 18g, Net Carbs: 13g, Fiber: 5g, Protein: 7g; Sodium: 347mg Macros: Fat: 65%, Carbs: 25%, Protein: 10%

## 177. Pesto Cauliflower SheetPan "Pizza

**Preparation Time: 15 Minutes**
**Cooking Time:** 25 Minutes
**Servings: 3**
**Ingredients:**
1 head cauliflower, trimmed
1/4 cup extravirgin olive oil
1 teaspoon salt
1/2 teaspoon freshly ground black pepper
1 teaspoon garlic powder
4 tablespoons Arugula and Walnut Pesto or storebought pesto
1 cup shredded wholemilk mozzarella or Italian cheese blend
1/2 cup crumbled feta cheese
**Directions:**
Preheat the oven to 425°F.

Remove the stem and bottom leaves from a head of cauliflower and carefully break into large florets—the larger, the better. Thinly slice each floret from top to stem to about 1/4inch thickness.

Line a large rimmed baking sheet with aluminum foil and drizzle with the olive oil, spreading the oil around with your fingers to coat the foil. Lay the cauliflower out in a single layer on the oiled sheet. Sprinkle with salt, pepper, and garlic powder.

Place in the oven and roast until softened, 15 to 20 minutes. Remove from the oven and spread the pesto evenly over top of the cauliflower. Sprinkle with the shredded cheese and feta, return to the oven, and roast for 10 more minutes, or until the cheese is melted and the cauliflower is soft.

Turn the broiler to low and broil until browned and bubbly on top, 3 to 5 minutes. Remove from the oven, allow to cool slightly, and cut into large squares to serve.
**Nutrition:**
Calories: 346,
Total Fat: 30g,
Total Carbs: 7g,
Net Carbs: 5g,
Fiber: 2g,
Protein: 12g;
Sodium: 938mg
Macros: Fat: 78%, Carbs: 8%, Protein: 14%

## 178. Greek Stewed Zucchini
**Preparation Time: 15 Minutes**
**Cooking Time:** 25 Minutes
**Servings: 3**
**Ingredients:**
1/4 cup extravirgin olive oil
1 small yellow onion, peeled and slivered
4 medium zucchini squash, cut into 1/2inchthick rounds
4 small garlic cloves, minced
1 to 2 teaspoons dried oregano
2 cups chopped tomatoes
1/2 cup halved and pitted Kalamata olives
3/4 cup crumbled feta cheese
1/4 cup chopped fresh flatleaf Italian parsley, for garnish (optional)
**Directions:**
In a large skillet, heat the oil over mediumhigh heat. Add the slivered onion and sauté until just tender, 6 to 8 minutes. Add the zucchini, garlic, and oregano and sauté another 6 to 8 minutes, or until zucchini is just tender. 2.Add the tomatoes and bring to a boil. Reduce the heat to low and add the olives. Cover and simmer on low heat for 20 minutes, or until the flavors

have developed and the zucchini is
very tender.

3.Serve warm topped with feta and parsley (if using).

**Nutrition:**
Calories: 272,
Total Fat: 20g,
Total Carbs: 15g,
Net Carbs: 10g,
Fiber: 5g,
Protein: 8g;

# CHAPTER 13:

# Salad Recipes

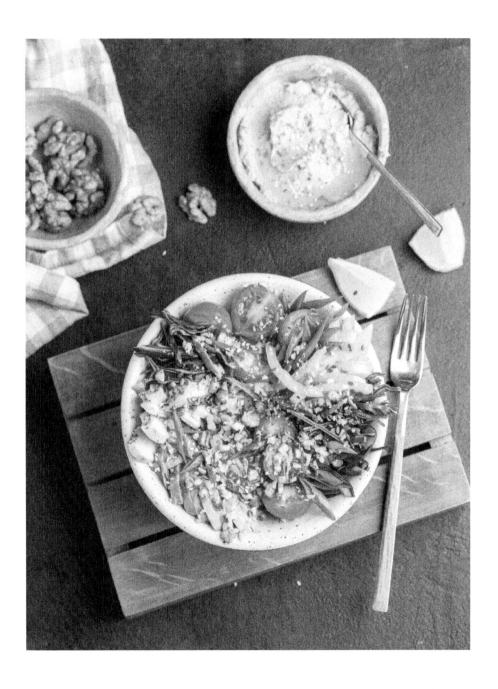

## 179. Cauliflower Tabbouleh Salad

**Preparation Time: 15 Minutes**
**Cooking Time:** 5 Minutes
**Servings: 3**
**Ingredients:**
6 tablespoons extravirgin olive oil, divided
4 cups riced cauliflower
3 garlic cloves, finely minced
11/2 teaspoons salt
1/2 teaspoon freshly ground black pepper
1/2 large cucumber, peeled, seeded, and chopped
1/2 cup chopped mint leaves
1/2 cup chopped Italian parsley
1/2 cup chopped pitted Kalamata olives
2 tablespoons minced red onion
Juice of 1 lemon (about 2 tablespoons)
2 cups baby arugula or spinach leaves
2 medium avocados, peeled, pitted, and diced
1 cup quartered cherry tomatoes
**Directions:**
In a large skillet, heat 2 tablespoons of olive oil over mediumhigh heat. Add the riced cauliflower, garlic, salt, and pepper and sauté until just tender but not mushy, 3 to 4 minutes. Remove from the heat and place in a large bowl.

Add the cucumber, mint, parsley, olives, red onion, lemon juice, and remaining 4 tablespoons olive oil and toss well. Place in the refrigerator, uncovered, and refrigerate for at least 30 minutes, or up to 2 hours.
Before serving, add the arugula, avocado, and tomatoes and toss to combine well. Season to taste with salt and pepper and serve cold or at room temperature.

**Nutrition:**
Calories: 235
Fat: 21g
Protein: 4g
Carbs: 12g
Fiber: 6g
Sodium: 623mg

## 180. Beet Summer Salad

**Preparation Time: 15 Minutes**
**Cooking Time:** 40 Minutes
**Servings: 6**
**Ingredients:**
6 medium to large fresh red or yellow beets
1/3 cup plus 1 tablespoon extravirgin olive oil, divided
4 heads of Treviso radicchio
2 shallots, peeled and sliced
1/4 cup lemon juice
1/2 teaspoon salt
6 ounces (170 g) feta cheese, crumbled
**Directions:**
Preheat the oven to 400°F (205°C).
Cut off the stems and roots of the beets. Wash the beets thoroughly and dry them off with a paper towel.
Peel the beets using a vegetable peeler. Cut into 1/2inch pieces and put them into a large bowl.
Add 1 tablespoon of olive oil to the bowl and toss to coat, then pour the beets out onto a baking sheet. Spread the beets so that they are evenly distributed.
Bake for 35 to 40 minutes until the beets are tender, turning once or twice with a spatula.
When the beets are done cooking, set them aside and let cool for 10 minutes. While the beets are cooling, cut the radicchio into 1inch pieces and place on a serving dish.

Once the beets have cooled, spoon them over the radicchio, then evenly distribute the shallots over the beets.

In a small bowl, whisk together the remaining 1/3 cup of olive oil, lemon juice, and salt. Drizzle the layered salad with dressing. Finish off the salad with feta cheese on top.

**Nutrition:**
Calories: 389
Fat: 31g
Protein: 10g
Carbs: 22g
Fiber: 5g
Sodium: 893mg

## 181. Tomato and Lentil Salad with Feta

**Preparation Time: 15 Minutes**
**Cooking Time:** 30 Minutes
**Servings: 3**
**Ingredients:**
3 cups water
1 cup brown or green lentils, picked over and rinsed
11/2 teaspoons salt, divided
2 large ripe tomatoes
2 Persian cucumbers
1/3 cup lemon juice
1/2 cup extravirgin olive oil
1 cup crumbled feta cheese
**Directions:**
In a large pot over medium heat, bring the water, lentils, and 1 teaspoon of salt to a simmer, then reduce heat to low. Cover the pot and continue to cook, stirring occasionally, for 30 minutes. (The lentils should be cooked so that they no longer have a crunch, but still hold their form. You should be able to smooth the lentil between your two fingers when pinched.)

Once the lentils are done cooking, strain them to remove any excess water and put them into a large bowl. Let cool.

Dice the tomatoes and cucumbers, then add them to the lentils.

In a small bowl, whisk together the lemon juice, olive oil, and remaining 1/2 teaspoon salt.

Pour the dressing over the lentils and vegetables. Add the feta cheese to the bowl, and gently toss all of the ingredients together.

**Nutrition:**
Calories: 521
Fat: 36g
Protein: 18g
Carbs: 35g
Fiber: 15g
Sodium: 1304mg

## 182. Quinoa and Garbanzo Salad

**Preparation Time: 15 Minutes**
**Cooking Time:** 25 Minutes
**Servings: 3**
**Ingredients:**
4 cups water
2 cups red or yellow quinoa
2 teaspoons salt, divided
1 cup thinly sliced onions (red or white)
1 (16ounce / 454g) can garbanzo beans, rinsed and drained
1/3 cup extravirgin olive oil
1/4 cup lemon juice
1 teaspoon freshly ground black pepper
**Directions:**
In a 3quart pot over medium heat, bring the water to a boil.

Add the quinoa and 1 teaspoon of salt to the pot. Stir, cover, and let cook over low heat for 15 to 20 minutes.

Turn off the heat, fluff the quinoa with a fork, cover again, and let stand for 5 to 10 more minutes.

Put the cooked quinoa, onions, and garbanzo beans in a large bowl.

In a separate small bowl, whisk together the olive oil, lemon juice, remaining 1 teaspoon of salt, and black pepper.

Add the dressing to the quinoa mixture and gently toss everything together. Serve warm or cold.

**Nutrition:**
Calories: 318
Fat: 6g
Protein: 9g
Carbs: 43g
Fiber: 13g
Sodium: 585mg

## 183. Winter Salad with Red Wine Vinaigrette

**Preparation Time: 15 Minutes**
**Cooking Time:** 25 Minutes
**Servings: 3**
**Ingredients:**
1 small green apple, thinly sliced
6 stalks kale, stems removed and greens roughly chopped
1/2 cup crumbled feta cheese
1/2 cup dried currants
1/2 cup chopped pitted Kalamata olives
1/2 cup thinly sliced radicchio
2 scallions, both green and white parts, thinly sliced
1/4 cup peeled, julienned carrots
2 celery stalks, thinly sliced
1/4 cup Red Wine Vinaigrette
Salt and freshly ground black pepper, to taste (optional)
**Directions:**
In a large bowl, combine the apple, kale, feta, currants, olives, radicchio, scallions, carrots, and celery and mix well. Drizzle with the vinaigrette. Season with salt and pepper (if using), then serve.

**Nutrition:**
Calories: 253 Fat: 15g
Protein: 6g Carbs: 29g
Fiber: 4g Sodium: 480mg

## 184. Avocado and Hearts of Palm Salad

**Preparation Time: 15 Minutes**
**Cooking Time:** 25 Minutes
**Servings: 3**
**Ingredients:**
2 (14ounce / 397g) cans hearts of palm, drained and cut into 1/2inchthick slices
1 avocado, cut into 1/2inch pieces
1 cup halved yellow cherry tomatoes
1/2 small shallot, thinly sliced
1/4 cup coarsely chopped flatleaf parsley
2 tablespoons lowfat mayonnaise
2 tablespoons extravirgin olive oil
1/4 teaspoon salt
1/8 teaspoon freshly ground black pepper
**Directions:**
In a large bowl, toss the hearts of palm, avocado, tomatoes, shallot, and parsley.

In a small bowl, whisk the mayonnaise, olive oil, salt, and pepper, then mix into the large bowl.
**Nutrition:**
Calories: 192
Fat: 15g
Protein: 5g Carbs: 14g
Fiber: 7g
Sodium: 841mg

## 185. Arugula and Walnut Salad

**Preparation Time: 15 Minutes**
**Cooking Time:**
**Servings: 7**
**Ingredients:**
4 tablespoons extravirgin olive oil

Zest and juice of 2 clementines or 1 orange (2 to 3 tablespoons)
1 tablespoon red wine vinegar
1/2 teaspoon salt
1/4 teaspoon freshly ground black pepper
8 cups baby arugula
1 cup coarsely chopped walnuts
1 cup crumbled goat cheese
1/2 cup pomegranate seeds

**Directions:**

In a small bowl, whisk together the olive oil, zest and juice, vinegar, salt, and pepper and set aside.

To assemble the salad for serving, in a large bowl, combine the arugula, walnuts, goat cheese, and pomegranate seeds. Drizzle with the dressing and toss to coat.

**Nutrition:**
Calories: 444
Fat: 40g
Protein: 10g
Carbs: 11g
Fiber: 3g
Sodium: 412mg

## 186. Kale Salad with Anchovy Dressing

**Preparation Time: 15 Minutes**
**Cooking Time: 0**
**Servings: 7**
**Ingredients:**
1 large bunch lacinato or dinosaur kale
1/4 cup toasted pine nuts
1 cup shaved or coarsely shredded fresh Parmesan cheese
1/4 cup extravirgin olive oil
8 anchovy fillets, roughly chopped
2 to 3 tablespoons freshly squeezed lemon juice (from 1 large lemon)
2 teaspoons red pepper flakes (optional)

**Directions:**

Remove the rough center stems from the kale leaves and roughly tear each leaf into about 4by1inch strips. Place the torn kale in a large bowl and add the pine nuts and cheese.

In a small bowl, whisk together the olive oil, anchovies, lemon juice, and red pepper flakes (if using). Drizzle over the salad and toss to coat well. Let sit at room temperature 30 minutes before serving, tossing again just prior to serving.

**Nutrition:**
Calories: 337
Fat: 25g
Protein: 16g
Carbs: 12g
Fiber: 2g
Sodium: 603mg

## 187. Authentic Greek Salad

**Preparation Time: 15 Minutes**
**Cooking Time: 0**
**Servings: 3**
**Ingredients:**
2 large English cucumbers
4 Roma tomatoes, quartered
1 green bell pepper, cut into 1 to 11/2inch chunks
1/4 small red onion, thinly sliced
4 ounces (113 g) pitted Kalamata olives
1/4 cup extravirgin olive oil
2 tablespoons freshly squeezed lemon juice
1 tablespoon red wine vinegar
1 tablespoon chopped fresh oregano or 1 teaspoon dried oregano
1/4 teaspoon freshly ground black pepper
4 ounces (113 g) crumbled traditional feta cheese

**Directions:**

Cut the cucumbers in half lengthwise and then into 1/2inchthick halfmoons. Place in a large bowl.

Add the quartered tomatoes, bell pepper, red onion, and olives.
In a small bowl, whisk together the olive oil, lemon juice, vinegar, oregano, and pepper. Drizzle over the vegetables and toss to coat.

Divide between salad plates and top each with 1 ounce (28 g) of feta.

**Nutrition:**
Calories: 278
Fat: 22g
Protein: 8g
Carbs: 12g
Fiber: 4g
Sodium: 572mg

## 188. Israeli Salad

**Preparation Time: 15 Minutes**
**Cooking Time:** 5 Minutes
**Servings: 5**
**Ingredients:**
1/4 cup pine nuts
1/4 cup shelled pistachios
1/4 cup coarsely chopped walnuts
1/4 cup shelled pumpkin seeds
1/4 cup shelled sunflower seeds
2 large English cucumbers, unpeeled and finely chopped
1 pint cherry tomatoes, finely chopped
1/2 small red onion, finely chopped
1/2 cup finely chopped fresh flatleaf Italian parsley
1/4 cup extravirgin olive oil
2 to 3 tablespoons freshly squeezed lemon juice (from 1 lemon)
1 teaspoon salt
1/4 teaspoon freshly ground black pepper
4 cups baby arugula
**Directions:**
In a large dry skillet, toast the pine nuts, pistachios, walnuts, pumpkin seeds, and sunflower seeds over mediumlow heat until golden and fragrant, 5 to 6 minutes, being careful not to burn them. Remove from the heat and set aside.
In a large bowl, combine the cucumber, tomatoes, red onion, and parsley.

In a small bowl, whisk together olive oil, lemon juice, salt, and pepper. Pour over the chopped vegetables and toss to coat.
Add the toasted nuts and seeds and arugula and toss with the salad to blend well. Serve at room temperature or chilled.

**Nutrition:**
Calories: 414
Fat: 34g
Protein: 10g
Carbs: 17g
Fiber: 6g
Sodium: 642mg

## 189. *Arugula Salad*

**Preparation Time: 15 Minutes**
**Cooking Time:** 0
**Servings: 6**
**Ingredients:**
4 cups arugula leaves
1 cup cherry tomatoes
1/4 cup pine nuts
1 tbsp. rice vinegar
2 tbsp. olive/grapeseed oil
.25 cup grated parmesan cheese
Black pepper & salt (as desired)
1 large sliced avocado
**Directions:**
Peel and slice the avocado.
Rinse and dry the arugula leaves, grate the cheese, and slice the cherry tomatoes into halves.
Combine the arugula, pine nuts, tomatoes, oil, vinegar, salt, pepper, and cheese.
Toss the salad to mix and portion it onto plates with the avocado slices to serve.
Serve.
**Nutrition:**
Calories: 257
Fat: 23 g
Protein: 6.1 g

## 190. Chickpea Salad
**Preparation Time: 15 Minutes**
**Cooking Time:** 0
**Servings: 3**
**Ingredients:**
15 oz. cooked chickpeas
1 diced Roma tomato
1/2 of 1 diced green medium bell pepper
1 tbsp. fresh parsley
1 small white onion
5 tsp. minced garlic
1 lemon juiced
**Directions:**
Chop the tomato, green pepper, and onion.
Mince the garlic.
Combine each of the fixings into a salad bowl and toss well.
Cover the salad to chill for at least 15 minutes in the fridge.
Serve when ready.
**Nutrition:**
Calories: 163
Fat: 7 g
Protein: 4 g

## 191. Chopped Israeli Mediterranean Pasta Salad
**Preparation Time: 15 Minutes**
**Cooking Time:** 14 Minutes
**Servings: 4**
**Ingredients:**
5 lb. small bow tie or other small pasta
1/3 cup Cucumber
1/3 cup Radish
1/3 cup Tomato
1/3 cup yellow bell pepper
1/3 cup orange bell pepper
1/3 cup Black olives
1/3 cup Green olives
1/3 cup Red onions
1/3 cup Pepperoncini
1/3 cup Feta cheese
1/3 cup fresh thyme leaves
(1 tsp.) dried oregano
Dressing:
0.25 cup + more, olive oil
1 lemon juice
**Directions:**
Slice the green olives into halves.
Dice the feta and pepperoncini and finely dice the remainder of the veggies.

Prepare a pot of water with the salt and simmer the pasta until it's "Al dente" (checking at two minutes under the listed time).
Rinse and drain in cold water.
Combine a small amount of oil with the pasta.
Add the salt, pepper, oregano, thyme, and veggies.
Pour in the rest of the oil, lemon juice, and mix and fold in the grated feta.
Pop it into the fridge within two hours, best if overnight.
Taste test and adjust the seasonings to your liking.
Add fresh thyme.
Serve.
**Nutrition:**
Calories: 65
Fat: 5.6 g
Protein: 0.8 g

## 192. Feta Tomato Salad
**Preparation Time: 15 Minutes**
**Cooking Time:** 0
**Servings: 3**
**Ingredients:**
2 tbsp. balsamic vinegar
5 tsp. freshly minced basil (1.5 tsp.) or dried
5 tsp. salt
5 cup coarsely chopped sweet onion
2 tbsp. Olive oil
1 lb. cherry or grape tomatoes

25 cup crumbled feta cheese
**Directions:**
Whisk the salt, basil, and vinegar.
Toss the onion into the vinegar mixture for 5 minutes
Slice the tomatoes into halves and stir in the tomatoes, feta cheese, and oil to serve.
Serve.
**Nutrition:**
Calories: 121
Fat: 9 g
Protein: 3 g

## 193. Greek Pasta Salad
**Preparation Time: 15 Minutes**
**Cooking Time:** 0
**Servings: 3**
**Ingredients:**
1 cup penne pasta
1.5 tsp. lemon juice
2 tbsp. red wine vinegar
1 garlic clove
1 tsp. dried oregano
Black pepper and sea salt (as desired)
1.33 cup olive oil
5 halved cherry tomatoes
1/2 of 1 small red onion
1/2 of 1 green & red bell pepper each
1/4 of 1 cucumber
.25 cup black olives
.25 cup crumbled feta cheese
**Directions:**
Slice the cucumber and olives.
Chop/dice the onion, peppers, and garlic and slice the tomatoes into halves.
Arrange a large pot with water and salt using the hightemperature setting.
Once it's boiling, add the pasta and cook for 11 minutes.
Rinse it using cold water and drain it in a colander.
Whisk the oil, juice, salt, pepper, vinegar, oregano, and garlic.

Combine the cucumber, cheese, olives, peppers, pasta, onions, and tomatoes in a large salad dish.
Add the vinaigrette over the pasta and toss.
Chill in the fridge (covered) for about 3 hours and serve as desired.
Serve.
**Nutrition:**
Calories: 307
Fat: 23.6 g
Protein: 5.4 g

## 194. Apples and Pomegranate Salad
**Preparation Time: 15 Minutes**
**Cooking Time:** 0
**Servings: 8**
**Ingredients:**
3 big apples, cored and cubed
1 cup pomegranate seeds
3 cups baby arugula
1 cup walnuts, chopped
1 tbsp. olive oil
1 tsp. white sesame seeds
2 tbsp. apple cider vinegar
**Directions:**
Mix the apples with the arugula and the rest of the ingredients in a bowl,
Toss and serve cold.
Serve.
**Nutrition:**
Calories: 160
Fat: 4.3 g
Protein: 10 g

## 195. Pork and Greens Salad
**Preparation Time: 15 Minutes**
**Cooking Time:** 45 Minutes
**Servings: 3**
**Ingredients:**
1pound pork chops
8 ounces white mushrooms, sliced
1/2 cup Italian dressing
6 cups mixed salad greens

6 ounces jarred artichoke hearts, drained

Salt and black pepper to the taste

1/2 cup basil, chopped

1 tbsp. olive oil

**Directions:**

Heat a pan with the oil over mediumhigh heat, add the pork, and brown for 5 minutes.

Add the mushrooms, stir and sauté for 5 minutes more.

Add the dressing, artichokes, salad greens, salt, pepper, and basil, cook for 45 minutes, divide everything into bowls.

Serve.

**Nutrition:**

Calories: 235

Fat: 5 g

Protein: 11 g

## 196. Creamy Chicken Salad

**Preparation Time: 15 Minutes**

**Cooking Time:** 0

**Servings: 3**

**Ingredients:**

20 ounces chicken meat

1/2 cup pecans, chopped

1 cup green grapes

1/2 cup celery, chopped

2 ounces canned mandarin oranges, drained

For the Creamy Cucumber Salad Dressing:

1 cup Greek yogurt cucumber, chopped garlic clove

1 tsp. lemon juice

**Directions:**

Mix all the ingredients

**Nutrition:**

Calories: 2305

Protein: 5.3 g

Fat: 62 g

## 197. Cheese Beet Salad

**Preparation Time: 15 Minutes**

**Cooking Time:** 0

**Servings: 3**

**Ingredients:**

6 red beets

3 ounces feta cheese

2 tbsp. olive oil

2 tbsp. balsamic vinegar

**Directions:**

Combine everything together. Serve.

**Nutrition:**

Calories: 230

Protein: 7.3 g

Fat: 12 g

## 198. Melon Salad

**Preparation Time: 15 Minutes**

**Cooking Time:** 0

**Servings: 4**

**Ingredients:**

1/4 tsp. sea salt

1/4 tsp. black pepper

1 tbsp. balsamic vinegar

1 cantaloupe

1cup watermelons

2 cups mozzarella balls, fresh

1/3 cup basil, fresh & torn

2 tbsp. olive oil

**Directions:**

Spoon out balls of cantaloupe, then situate them in a colander over a bowl.

Using a melon baller to cut the watermelon as well.

Drain fruits for ten minutes, then chill the juice.

Wipe the bowl dry and then place your fruit in it.

Mix in basil, oil, vinegar, mozzarella, and tomatoes before seasoning and gently mix.

Serve.
**Nutrition:**
Calories: 218
Protein: 10 g
Fat: 13 g

## 199. Chicken Oatmeal Soup
**Preparation Time: 10 minutes**
**Cooking Time: 15 minutes**
**Servings: 2**
**Ingredients:**
1 cup oats
4 cups of water
1 oz fresh dill, chopped
10 oz chicken fillet, chopped
1 teaspoon ground black pepper
1 teaspoon potato starch
1/2 carrot, diced
**Directions:**
Put the chopped chicken in the saucepan, add water and bring it to boil. Simmer the chicken for 10 minutes.
Add dill, ground black pepper, oats, and diced carrot.
Bring the soup to boil and add potato starch. Stir it until soup starts to thicken. Simmer the soup for 5 minutes on the low heat.
**Nutrition:**
192 calories,
19.8g protein,
16.1g carbohydrates,
5.5g fat,
2.7g fiber,
50mg cholesterol,
72mg sodium,

## 200. Celery Cream Soup
**Preparation Time: 10 minutes**
**Cooking Time: 25 minutes**
**Servings: 1**
**Ingredients:**
2 cups celery stalk, chopped
1 shallot, chopped

1 potato, chopped
4 cups low-sodium vegetable stock
1 tablespoon margarine
1 teaspoon white pepper
**Directions:**
Melt the margarine in the saucepan, add shallot, and celery stalk. Cook the vegetables for 5 minutes. Stir them occasionally.
After this, add vegetable stock and potato.
Simmer the soup for 15 minutes.
Blend the soup tilly ou get the creamy texture and sprinkle with white pepper. Simmer it for 5 minutes more.
**Nutrition:**
88 calories,
2.3g protein,
13.3g carbohydrates,
3g fat,
2.9g fiber,
0mg cholesterol,
217mg sodium,
449mg potassium.

## 201. Cauliflower Soup
**Preparation Time: 10 minutes**
**Cooking Time: 20 minutes**
**Servings: 2**
**Ingredients:**
1 cup cauliflower, chopped
1/4 cup potato, chopped
1 cup skim milk
1 cup of water
1 teaspoon ground coriander
1 teaspoon margarine
**Directions:**
Put cauliflower and potato in the saucepan.
Add water and boil the ingredients for 15 minutes.
Then add ground coriander and margarine.
With the help of the immersion blender, blend the soup until smooth.

Add skim milk and stir well.
**Nutrition:**
82 calories,
5.2g protein,
10.3g carbohydrates,
2g fat,
1.5g fiber,
2mg cholesterol,
106mg sodium,

## 202. Buckwheat Soup
**Preparation Time: 10 minutes**
**Cooking Time: 25 minutes**
**Servings: 2**
**Ingredients:**
1/2 cup buckwheat
1 carrot, chopped
1 yellow onion, diced
1 tablespoon avocado oil
1 tablespoon fresh dill, chopped
1-pound chicken breast, chopped
1 teaspoon ground black pepper
6 cups of water
**Directions:**
Saute the onion, carrot, and avocado oil in the saucepan for 5 minutes. Stir them from time to time.
Then add buckwheat, chicken breast, and ground black pepper.
Add water and close the lid.
Simmer the soup for 20 minutes.
After this, add dill and remove the soup from the heat. Leave it for 10 minutes to rest.
**Nutrition:**
152 calories, 18.4g protein,
13.5g carbohydrates,
2.7g fat, 2.3g fiber, 48mg cholesterol,
48mg sodium,

## 203. Spring Greens Salad
**Preparation Time: 15 Minutes**
**Cooking Time: 0 minutes**
**Servings: 2**
**Ingredients:**

1/2 cup radish, sliced
1 cup fresh spinach, chopped
1/2 cup green peas, cooked
1/2 lemon
1 cup arugula, chopped
1 tablespoon avocado oil
1/2 teaspoon dried sage
**Directions:**
In the salad bowl, mix up radish, spinach, green peas, arugula, and dried sage.
Then squeeze the lemon over the salad.

Add avocado oil and shake the salad.
**Nutrition:**
54 calories,
3.1g protein,
9g carbohydrates,
1.3g fat,
3.6g fiber,
0mg cholesterol,
28mg sodium,

## 204. Tuna Salad
**Preparation Time: 7 minutes**
**Cooking Time: 0 minutes**
**Servings: 2**
**Ingredients:**
1/2 cup low-fat Greek yogurt
8 oz tuna, canned
1/2 cup fresh parsley, chopped
1 cup corn kernels, cooked
1/2 teaspoon ground black pepper
**Directions:**
Mix up tuna, parsley, kernels, and ground black pepper.
Then add yogurt and stir the salad until it is homogenous.
**Nutrition:**
172 calories,
17.8g protein,
13.6g carbohydrates,
5.5g fat,
1.4g fiber,
19mg cholesterol,

55mg sodium,

## 205. Fish Salad
**Preparation Time: 15 Minutes**
**Cooking Time: 0 minutes**
**Servings: 2**
**Ingredients:**
7 oz canned salmon, shredded
1 tablespoon lime juice
1 tablespoon low-fat yogurt
1 cup baby spinach, chopped
1 teaspoon capers, drained and chopped
**Directions:**
Mix up all ingredients together and transfer them in the salad bowl.
**Nutrition:**
71 calories,
10.1g protein,
0.8g carbohydrates,
3.2g fat,
0.2g fiber,
22mg cholesterol,
52mg sodium,

## 206. Salmon Salad
**Preparation Time: 10 minutes**
**Cooking Time: 0 minutes**
**Servings: 2**
**Ingredients:**
4 oz canned salmon, flaked
1 tablespoon lemon juice
2 tablespoons red bell pepper, chopped
1 tablespoon red onion, chopped
1 teaspoon dill, chopped
1 tablespoon olive oil
**Directions:**
Mix up all ingredients in the salad bowl.

**Nutrition:**
119 calories,
8.3g protein,
6.6g carbohydrates,
7.3g fat,

1.2g fiber,
17mg cholesterol,
21mg sodium,

## 207. Arugula Salad with Shallot
**Preparation Time: 10 minutes**
**Cooking Time: 0 minutes**
**Servings: 2**
**Ingredients:**
1 cup cucumber, chopped
1 tablespoon lemon juice
1 tablespoon avocado oil
2 shallots, chopped
1/2 cup black olives, sliced
3 cups arugula, chopped
**Directions:**
Mix up all ingredients from the list above in the salad bowl and refrigerate in the fridge for 5 minutes.
**Nutrition:**
33 calories,
0.8g protein,
2.9g carbohydrates,
2.4g fat,
1.1g fiber,
0mg cholesterol,
152mg sodium,

## 208. Watercress Salad
**Preparation Time: 10 minutes**
**Cooking Time: 4 minutes**
**Servings: 2**
**Ingredients:**
2 cups asparagus, chopped
16 ounces shrimp, cooked
4 cups watercress, torn
1 tablespoon apple cider vinegar
1/4 cup olive oil
**Directions:**
In the mixing bowl mix up asparagus, shrimps, watercress, and olive oil.
**Nutrition:**
264 calories,
28.3g protein,

4.5g carbohydrates,
14.8g fat, 1.8g fiber,
239mg cholesterol,
300mg sodium,

## 209. Pumpkin Cream Soup
**Preparation Time: 10 minutes**
**Cooking Time: 20 minutes**
**Servings: 2**
**Ingredients:**
1-pound pumpkin, chopped
1 teaspoon ground cumin
1/2 cup cauliflower, chopped
4 cups of water
1 teaspoon ground turmeric
1/2 teaspoon ground nutmeg
1 tablespoon fresh dill, chopped
1 teaspoon olive oil
1/2 cup skim milk
**Directions:**
Roast the pumpkin with olive oil in the saucepan for 3 minutes.
Then stir well and add cauliflower, cumin, turmeric, nutmeg, and water.
Close the lid and cook the soup on medium mode for 15 minutes or until the pumpkin is soft.
Then blend the mixture until smooth and add skim milk. Remove the soup from heat and top with dill.
**Nutrition:**
56 calories,
2.2g protein,
10g carbohydrates,
1.4g fat,
3.1g fiber,
0mg cholesterol,
28mg sodium,

## 210. Zucchini Noodles Soup
**Preparation Time: 10 minutes**
**Cooking Time: 15 minutes**
**Servings: 2**
**Ingredients:**
2 zucchinis, trimmed

4 cups low-sodium chicken stock
2 oz fresh parsley, chopped
1/2 teaspoon chili flakes
1 oz carrot, shredded
1 teaspoon canola oil
**Directions:**
Roast the carrot with canola oil in the saucepan for 5 minutes over the medium-low heat.
Stir it well and add chicken stock. Bring the mixture to boil.
Meanwhile, make the noodles from the zucchini with the help of the spiralizer. Add them in the boiling soup liquid.
Add parsley and chili flakes. Bring the soup to boil and remove it from heat.
Leave for 10 minutes to rest.
**Nutrition:**
39 calories,
2.7g protein,
4.9g carbohydrates,
1.5g fat, 1.7g fiber,
0mg cholesterol,
158mg sodium,

## 211. Steamed Tomatoes Soup
**Preparation Time: 10 minutes**
**Cooking Time: 20 minutes**
**Servings: 1**
**Ingredients:**
2-pounds tomatoes
1/2 cup shallot, chopped
1 tablespoon avocado oil
1/2 teaspoon ground black pepper
1/4 teaspoon minced garlic
1 tablespoon dried basil
3 cups low-sodium chicken broth
**Directions:**
Cut the tomatoes into halves and Steam them in the preheated to 390F Steam for 1 minute from each side.
After this, transfer the Steamed

tomatoes in the blender and blend until smooth.

Place the shallot and avocado oil in the saucepan and roast it until light brown.

Add blended Steamed tomatoes, ground black pepper, and minced garlic.

Bring the soup to boil and sprinkle with dried basil.

Simmer the soup for 2 minutes more.

**Nutrition:**
72 calories,
4.1g protein,
13.4g carbohydrates,
0.9g fat,
3g fiber, 0mg cholesterol,
98mg sodium,

## 212. Sliced Mushrooms Salad
**Preparation Time: 10 minutes**
**Cooking Time: 20 minutes**
**Servings: 2**
**Ingredients:**
1 cup mushrooms, sliced
1 tablespoon margarine
1 cup lettuce, chopped
1 teaspoon lemon juice
1 tablespoon fresh dill, chopped
1 teaspoon cumin seeds
**Directions:**
Melt the margarine in the skillet.

Add mushrooms and lemon juice. Saute the vegetables for 20 minutes over the medium heat.

Then transfer the cooked mushrooms in the salad bowl, add lettuce, dill, and cumin seeds.

Stir the salad well.

**Nutrition:**
35 calories,
0.9g protein, 1.7g carbohydrates,
3.1g fat, 0.5g fiber, 0mg cholesterol,
38mg sodium,

## 213. Tender Green Beans Salad
**Preparation Time: 15 Minutes**
**Cooking Time: 5 minutes**
**Servings: 2**
**Ingredients:**
2 cups green beans, trimmed, chopped, cooked
2 tablespoons olive oil
2 pounds shrimp, cooked, peeled
1 cup tomato, chopped
1/4 cup apple cider vinegar
**Directions:**
Mix up all ingredients together.

Then transfer the salad in the salad bowl.

**Nutrition:**
179 calories, 26.5g protein,
4.6g carbohydrates, 5.5g fat,
1.2g fiber, 239mg cholesterol,
280mg sodium,

## 214. Crispy Fennel Salad
**Preparation Time: 15 Minutes**
**Cooking Time: 15 minutes**
**Servings: 2**
**Ingredients:**
1 fennel bulb, finely sliced
1 grapefruit, cut into segments
1 orange, cut into segments
2 tablespoons almond slices, toasted
1 teaspoon chopped mint
1 tablespoon chopped dill
Salt and pepper to taste
1 tablespoon grape seed oil
**Directions:**
Mix the fennel bulb with the grapefruit and orange segments on a platter.

Top with almond slices, mint and dill then drizzle with the oil and season with salt and pepper.

Serve the salad as fresh as possible.

**Nutrition:**
Calories:104 Fat:0.5g
Protein:3.1g Carbohydrates:25.5g

## 215. Red Beet Feta Salad

**Preparation Time: 15 Minutes**
**Cooking Time: 10 minutes**
**Servings: 2**
**Ingredients:**
6 red beets, cooked and peeled
3 oz. feta cheese, cubed
2 tablespoons extra virgin olive oil
2 tablespoons balsamic vinegar
**Directions:**
Combine the beets and feta cheese on a platter.
Drizzle with oil and vinegar and serve right away.
**Nutrition:**
Calories: 230
Fat: 12.0g
Protein: 7.3g
Carbohydrates: 26.3g

## 216. Cheesy Potato Mash

**Preparation Time: 15 Minutes**
**Cooking Time: 20 minutes**
**Servings: 2**
**Ingredients:**
2 pounds gold potatoes, peeled and cubed
1 and 1/2 cup cream cheese, soft
Sea salt and black pepper to the taste
1/2 cup almond milk
2 tablespoons chives, chopped
**Directions:**
Put potatoes in a pot, add water to cover, add a pinch of salt, bring to a simmer over medium heat, cook for 20 minutes, drain and mash them.
Add the rest of the ingredients except the chives and whisk well.
Add the chives, stir, divide between plates and serve as a side dish.
**Nutrition:**
calories 243
fat 14.2
fiber 1.4
carbs 3.5

protein 1.4

## 217. Provencal Summer Salad

**Preparation Time: 15 Minutes**
**Cooking Time: 25 minutes**
**Servings: 2**
**Ingredients:**
1 zucchini, sliced
1 eggplant, sliced
2 red onions, sliced
2 tomatoes, sliced
1 teaspoon dried mint
2 garlic cloves, minced
2 tablespoons balsamic vinegar
Salt and pepper to taste
**Directions:**
Season the zucchini, eggplant, onions and tomatoes with salt and pepper.
Cook the vegetable slices on the Steam until browned.
Transfer the vegetables in a salad bowl then add the mint, garlic and vinegar.
Serve the salad right away.
Nutrition:
Calories: 74
Fat: 0.5g
Protein: 3.0g
Carbohydrates: 16.5g

## 218. Sunflower Seeds And Arugula Garden Salad

**Preparation Time: 15 Minutes**
**Cooking Time: 10 minutes**
**Servings: 2**
**Ingredients:**
1/4 tsp black pepper
1/4 tsp salt
1 tsp fresh thyme, chopped
2 tbsp sunflower seeds, toasted
2 cups red grapes, halved
7 cups baby arugula, loosely packed
1 tbsp coconut oil
2 tsp honey
3 tbsp red wine vinegar

1/2 tsp stone-ground mustard

**Directions:**

In a small bowl, whisk together mustard, honey and vinegar. Slowly pour oil as you whisk.

In a large salad bowl, mix thyme, seeds, grapes and arugula.

Drizzle with dressing and serve.

**Nutrition:**
Calories per serving: 86.7
Protein: 1.6g
Carbs: 13.1g
Fat: 3.1g

## 219. Ginger Pumpkin Mash
**Preparation Time: 15 Minutes**
**Cooking Time: 30 minutes**
**Servings: 2**
**Ingredients:**
10 oz pumpkin, peeled
1/2 teaspoon butter
3/4 teaspoon ground ginger
1/3 teaspoon salt
**Directions:**
Chop the pumpkin into the cubes and bake in the preheated to the 360F oven for 30 minutes or until the pumpkin is soft.
After this, transfer the pumpkin cubes in the food processor.
Add butter, salt, and ground ginger.
Blend the vegetable until you get puree or use the potato masher for this step.
**Nutrition:**
calories 30
fat 0.7
fiber 2.1
carbs 6
protein 0.8

## 220. Yogurt Peppers Mix
**Preparation Time: 15 Minutes**
**Cooking Time: 10 minutes**
**Servings: 2**
**Ingredients:**
2 red bell peppers, cut into thick strips
2 tablespoons olive oil
3 shallots, chopped
3 garlic cloves, minced
Salt and black pepper to the taste
1/2 cup Greek yogurt
1 tablespoon cilantro, chopped

**Directions:**
Heat up a pan with the oil over medium heat, add the shallots and garlic, stir and cook for 5 minutes.
Add the rest of the ingredients, toss, cook for 10 minutes more, divide the mix between plates and serve as a side dish.
**Nutrition:**
calories 274
fat 11
fiber 3.5
protein 13.3
carbs 6.5

## 221. Lemony Carrots
**Preparation Time: 15 Minutes**
**Cooking Time: 40 minutes**
**Servings: 2**
**Ingredients:**
3 tablespoons olive oil
2 pounds baby carrots, trimmed
Salt and black pepper to the taste
1/2 teaspoon lemon zest, grated
1 tablespoon lemon juice
1/3 cup Greek yogurt
1 garlic clove, minced
1 teaspoon cumin, ground
1 tablespoon dill, chopped
**Directions:**
In a roasting pan, combine the carrots with the oil, salt, pepper and the rest of the ingredients except the dill, toss and bake at 400 degrees F for 20 minutes.
Reduce the temperature to 375 degrees F and cook for 20 minutes more.
Divide the mix between plates, sprinkle the dill on top and serve.
**Nutrition:**
calories 192
fat 5.4
fiber 3.4
carbs 7.3
protein 5.6

## 222. Roasted Vegetable Salad
**Preparation Time: 15 Minutes**
**Cooking Time: 30 minutes**
**Servings: 4**
**Ingredients:**
1/2 pound baby carrots
2 red onions, sliced
1 zucchini, sliced
2 eggplants, cubed
1 cauliflower, cut into florets
1 sweet potato, peeled and cubed
1 endive, sliced
3 tablespoons extra virgin olive oil
1 teaspoon dried basil
Salt and pepper to taste
1 lemon, juiced
1 tablespoon balsamic vinegar
**Directions:**
Combine the vegetables with the oil, basil, salt and pepper in a deep dish baking pan and cook in the preheated oven at 350F for 25-30 minutes.
When done, transfer in a salad bowl and add the lemon juice and vinegar. Serve the salad fresh.
**Nutrition:**
Calories:164
Fat:7.6g
Protein:3.7g
Carbohydrates:24.2g

## 223. Chicken Kale Soup
**Preparation Time: 15 Minutes**
**Cooking Time: 10 minutes**
**Servings: 2**
**Ingredients:**
2poundschicken breast, skinless
1/3cuponion
1tablespoonolive oil
14ounceschicken bone broth
1/2 cup olive oil
4 cups chicken stock
1/4 cup lemon juice
5ouncesbaby kale leaves
Salt, to taste

**Directions:**
Season chicken with salt and black pepper.
Heat olive oil over medium heat in a large skillet and add seasoned chicken.
Reduce the temperature and cook for about 15 minutes.
Shred the chicken and place in the crock pot.
Process the chicken broth and onions in a blender and blend until smooth.
Pour into crock pot and stir in the remaining ingredients.
Cook on low for about 6 hours, stirring once while cooking.
**Nutrition:**
Calories: 261
Carbs: 2g
Fats: 21g
Proteins: 14.1g
Sodium: 264mg
Sugar: 0.3g

## 224. Mozzarella Pasta Mix
**Preparation Time: 15 Minutes**
**Cooking Time: 15 minutes**
**Servings: 2**
**Ingredients:**
2 oz whole grain elbow macaroni
1 tablespoon fresh basil
1/4 cup cherry size Mozzarella
1/2 cup cherry tomatoes, halved
1 tablespoon olive oil
1 teaspoon dried marjoram
1 cup water, for cooking
**Directions:**
Boil elbow macaroni in water for 15 minutes. Drain water and chill macaroni little.
Chop fresh basil roughly and place it in the salad bowl.
Add Mozzarella, cherry tomatoes, dried marjoram, olive oil, amd macaroni.

Mix up salad well.
Nutrition:
calories 170 fat 9.7
fiber 1.1 carbs 15
protein 6

## 225. Quinoa Salad
**Preparation Time: 15 Minutes**
**Cooking Time: 20 minutes**
**Servings: 2**
**Ingredients:**
2 cups red quinoa
4 cups water
1 (15-oz.) can chickpeas, drained
1 medium red onion, chopped (1/2 cup)
3 TB. fresh mint leaves, finely chopped
1/4 cup extra-virgin olive oil
3 TB. fresh lemon juice
1/2 tsp. salt
1/2 tsp. fresh ground black pepper
**Directions:**
In a medium saucepan over medium-high heat, bring red quinoa and water to a boil. Cover, reduce heat to low, and cook for 20 minutes or until water is absorbed and quinoa is tender. Let cool.
In a large bowl, add quinoa, chickpeas, red onion, and mint.
In a small bowl, whisk together extra-virgin olive oil, lemon juice, salt, and black pepper. Pour dressing over quinoa mixture, and stir well to combine. Serve immediately, or refrigerate and enjoy for up to 2 or 3 days.

## 226. Couscous And Toasted Almonds
**Preparation Time: 15 Minutes**
**Cooking Time: 10 minutes**
**Servings: 2**
**Ingredients:**
1 cup (about 200 g) whole-grain couscous
400 ml boiling water
1 tablespoon extra-virgin olive oil
1/2 red onion, chopped
1/2 teaspoon ground ginger,
1/2 teaspoon ground cinnamon and
1/2 teaspoon ground coriander
2 tablespoons blanched almonds, toasted, and chopped
**Directions:**
Preheat the oven to 110C.
In a casserole, toss the couscous with the olive oil, onion, spices, salt and pepper. Stir in the boiling water, cover, and bake for 10 minutes. Fluff using a fork. Scatter the nuts over the top and then serve. Pair with harira.
Nutrition:
261.23 cal
8 g total fat
37 g carb
7 g protein
1 g sugar
6.85 mg sodium.

## 227. Spanish Tomato Salad
**Preparation Time: 15 Minutes**
**Cooking Time: 10 minutes**
**Servings: 2**
**Ingredients:**
1
pound tomatoes, cubed
2 cucumbers, cubed
2 garlic cloves, chopped
1 red onion, sliced
2 anchovy fillets
1 tablespoon balsamic vinegar
1 pinch chili powder
Salt and pepper to taste
**Directions:**
Combine the tomatoes, cucumbers, garlic and red onion in a bowl.
In a mortar, mix the anchovy fillets, vinegar, chili powder, salt and pepper.

Drizzle the mixture over the salad and mix well.

Serve the salad fresh.

**Nutrition**:
Calories: 61
Fat: 0.6g
Protein: 3.0g
Carbohydrates: 13.0g

## 228. Roasted Bell Pepper Salad With Anchovy Dressing

**Preparation Time: 15 Minutes**
**Cooking Time: 20 minutes**
**Servings: 2**
**Ingredients:**
8 roasted red bell peppers, sliced
2 tablespoons pine nuts
1 cup cherry tomatoes, halved
2 tablespoons chopped parsley
4 anchovy fillets
1 lemon, juiced
1 garlic clove
1 tablespoon extra-virgin olive oil
Salt and pepper to taste
**Directions:**
Combine the anchovy fillets, lemon juice, garlic and olive oil in a mortar and mix them well.

Mix the rest of the ingredients in a salad bowl then drizzle in the dressing.

Serve the salad as fresh as possible.

**Nutrition:**
Calories: 81
Fat: 7.0g
Protein: 2.4g
Carbohydrates: 4.0g

## 229. Warm Shrimp And Arugula Salad

**Preparation Time: 15 Minutes**
**Cooking Time: 20 minutes**
**Servings: 2**
**Ingredients:**
2 tablespoons extra virgin olive oil

2 garlic cloves, minced

1 red pepper, sliced
1 pound fresh shrimps, peeled and deveined
1 orange, juiced
Salt and pepper to taste
3 cups arugula
**Directions:**
Heat the oil in a frying pan and stir in the garlic and red pepper. Cook for 1 minute then add the shrimps.

Cook for 5 minutes then add the orange juice and cook for another 5 more minutes.

When done, spoon the shrimps and the sauce over the arugula.

Serve the salad fresh.

Nutrition:
Calories:232
Fat:9.2g
Protein:27.0g
Carbohydrates:10.0g

## 230. Cheesy Tomato Salad

**Preparation Time: 15 Minutes**
**Cooking Time: 0 minutes**
**Servings: 2**
**Ingredients:**
2 pounds tomatoes, sliced
1 red onion, chopped
Sea salt and black pepper to the taste
4 ounces feta cheese, crumbled
2 tablespoons mint, chopped
A drizzle of olive oil
**Directions:**
In a salad bowl, mix the tomatoes with the onion and the rest of the ingredients, toss and serve as a side salad.

**Nutrition:**
calories 190
fat 4.5
fiber 3.4
carbs 8.7

protein 3.3

## 231. Garlic Cucumber Mix

**Preparation Time: 15 Minutes**
**Cooking Time: 10 minutes**
**Servings: 2**
**Ingredients:**
2 cucumbers, sliced
2 spring onions, chopped
2 tablespoons olive oil
3 garlic cloves, grated
1 tablespoon thyme, chopped
Salt and black pepper to the taste
3 and 1/2 ounces goat cheese, crumbled

**Directions:**
In a salad bowl, mix the cucumbers with the onions and the rest of the ingredients, toss and serve after keeping it in the fridge for 15 minutes.

**Nutrition:**
calories 140
fat 5.4
fiber 4.3
carbs 6.5
protein 4.8

## 232. Cucumber Salad Japanese Style

**Preparation Time: 15 Minutes**
**Cooking Time: 10 minutes**
**Servings: 2**
**Ingredients:**
1 1/2 tsp minced fresh ginger root
1 tsp salt
1/3 cup rice vinegar
2 large cucumbers, ribbon cut
4 tsp white sugar

**Directions:**
Mix well ginger, salt, sugar and vinegar in a small bowl.
Add ribbon cut cucumbers and mix well.
Let stand for at least one hour in the ref before serving.

**Nutrition:**
Calories 29

Fat: .2g
Protein: .7g
Carbs: 6.1g

## 233. Cheesy Keto Zucchini Soup

**Preparation Time: 15 Minutes**
**Cooking Time: 10 minutes**
**Servings: 2**
**Ingredients:**
1/2 medium onion, peeled and chopped
1 cup bone broth
1 tablespoon coconut oil
11/2 zucchinis, cut into chunks
1/2 tablespoon nutrition al yeast
Dash of black pepper
1/2 tablespoon parsley, chopped, for garnish
1/2 tablespoon coconut cream, for garnish

**Directions:**
Melt the coconut oil in a large pan over medium heat and add onions.
Sauté for about 3 minutes and add zucchinis and bone broth.
Reduce the heat to simmer for about 15 minutes and cover the pan.
Add nutrition al yeast and transfer to an immersion blender.
Blend until smooth and season with black pepper.
Top with coconut cream and parsley to serve.

**Nutrition:**
Calories: 154 Carbs: 8.9g Fats: 8.1g
Proteins: 13.4g Sodium: 93mg
Sugar: 3.9g

## 234. Steamed Salmon Summer Salad

**Preparation Time: 15 Minutes**
**Cooking Time: 30 minutes**
**Servings: 2**
**Ingredients:**

Salmon fillets - 2
Salt and pepper - to taste
Vegetable stock - 2 cups
Bulgur - 1 2 cup
Cherry tomatoes - 1 cup, halved
Sweet corn - 1 2 cup
Lemon - 1, juiced
Green olives - 1 2 cup, sliced
Cucumber - 1, cubed
Green onion - 1, chopped
Red pepper - 1, chopped
Red bell pepper - 1, cored and diced

**Directions:**
Heat a Steam pan on medium and then place salmon on, seasoning with salt and pepper. Steam both sides of salmon until brown and set aside.
Heat stock in sauce pan until hot and then add in bulgur and cook until liquid is completely soaked into bulgur. Mix salmon, bulgur and all other Ingredients in a salad bowl and again add salt and pepper, if desired, to suit your taste.
Serve salad as soon as completed.

**Nutrition:**
Calories 69
Fat 6.5 g
Fiber 2.6 g
Carbs 10.6 g
Protein 9.4 g

## 235. Dill Beets Salad

**Preparation Time: 15 Minutes**
**Cooking Time: 0 minutes**
**Servings: 2**
**Ingredients:**
2 pounds beets, cooked, peeled and cubed
2 tablespoons olive oil
1 tablespoon lemon juice
2 tablespoons balsamic vinegar
1 cup feta cheese, crumbled
3 small garlic cloves, minced
4 green onions, chopped

5 tablespoons parsley, chopped
Salt and black pepper to the taste
**Directions:**
In a bowl, mix the beets with the oil, lemon juice and the rest of the ingredients, toss and serve as a side dish.

**Nutrition:**
calories 268
fat 15.5
fiber 5.1
carbs 25.7
protein 9.6

## 236. Green Couscous With Broad Beans, Pistachio, And Dill

**Preparation Time: 15 Minutes**
**Cooking Time: 10 minutes**
**Servings: 2**
**Ingredients:**
200 g fresh or frozen broad beans, podded
2 teaspoons ground ginger
2 tablespoons spring onion, thinly sliced
2 tablespoons pistachio kernels, roughly chopped
2 tablespoons lemon juice, and wedges to serve
Dill, chopped - 1/4 cup
Olive oil, extra-virgin - 1/4 cup (about 60 ml)
1/2 onion, thinly sliced
Watercress, leaves picked - 1/2 bunch
1/2 avocado, chopped
1 green bell pepper, thinly sliced
1 garlic clove, crushed
1 cup (about 200 g) whole-grain couscous
1 1/2 cups boiling water
**Directions:**
In a heat-safe bowl, toss the couscous with the ginger and the onion. Stir in

the boiling water, cover and let stand for 5 minutes.

Meanwhile, cook the beans for about 3 minutes in boiling salted water, drain, and refresh under running cold water; discard the outer skins.

With a fork, fluff the couscous. Add the beans, avocado, bell pepper, spring onion, and dill.

In a bowl, whisk the olive oil, lemon juice, and garlic; toss with the couscous. Scatter the pistachio over the mix, serve with cress and the lemon wedges.

**Nutrition:**
608 calories
25.40 g total fat
51.50 g carb
18.10 g protein
45 mg sodium
 11 g fiber

## 237. Bell Peppers Salad

**Preparation Time: 15 Minutes**
**Cooking Time: 10 minutes**
**Servings: 2**
**Ingredients:**
2 green bell peppers, cut into thick strips
2 red bell peppers, cut into thick strips
2 tablespoons olive oil
1 garlic clove, minced
1/2 cup goat cheese, crumbled
A pinch of salt and black pepper
**Directions:**
In a bowl, mix the bell peppers with the garlic and the other ingredients, toss and serve.
**Nutrition:**
calories 193 fat 4.5
fiber 2 carbs 4.3
protein 3

## 238. Thyme Corn And Cheese Mix

**Preparation Time: 15 Minutes**

**Cooking Time: 10 minutes**
**Servings: 2**
**Ingredients:**
1 tablespoon olive oil
1 teaspoon thyme, chopped
1 cup scallions, sliced
2 cups corn
Salt and black pepper to the taste
2 tablespoons blue cheese, crumbled
1 tablespoon chives, chopped
**Directions:**
In a salad bowl, combine the corn with scallions, thyme and the rest of the ingredients, toss, divide between plates and serve.
**Nutrition:**
 calories 183
fat 5.5
fiber 7.5
carbs 14.5

## 239. Garden Salad With Oranges And Olives

**Preparation Time: 15 Minutes**
**Cooking Time: 10 minutes**
**Servings: 2**
**Ingredients:**
1/2 cup red wine vinegar
1 tbsp extra virgin olive oil
1 tbsp finely chopped celery
1 tbsp finely chopped red onion
16 large ripe black olives
2 garlic cloves
2 navel oranges, peeled and segmented
4 boneless, skinless chicken breasts, 4-oz each
4 garlic cloves, minced
8 cups leaf lettuce, washed and dried
Cracked black pepper to taste
**Directions:**
Preparation are the dressing by mixing pepper, celery, onion, olive oil, garlic and vinegar in a small bowl. Whisk well to combine.

Lightly grease grate and preheat Steam to high.

Rub chicken with the garlic cloves and discard garlic.

Steam chicken for 5 minutes per side or until cooked through.

Remove from Steam and let it stand for 5 minutes before cutting into 1/2-inch strips.

In 4 serving plates, evenly arrange two cups lettuce, 1/4 of the sliced oranges and 4 olives per plate.

Top each plate with 1/4 serving of Steamed chicken, evenly drizzle with dressing, serve and enjoy.

**Nutrition:**
Calories: 259.8 Protein: 48.9g
Carbs: 12.9g Fat: 1.4g

## 240. Smoked Salmon Lentil Salad

**Preparation Time: 15 Minutes**
**Cooking Time: 10 minutes**
**Servings: 2**
**Ingredients:**
1 cup green lentils, rinsed
2 cups vegetable stock
1/2 cup chopped parsley
2 tablespoons chopped cilantro
1 red pepper, chopped
1 red onion, chopped
Salt and pepper to taste
4 oz. smoked salmon, shredded
1 lemon, juiced
**Directions:**
Combine the lentils and stock in a saucepan. Cook on low heat for 15-20 minutes or until all the liquid has been absorbed completely.

Transfer the lentils in a salad bowl and add the parsley, cilantro, red pepper and onion. Season with salt and pepper.

Add the smoked salmon and lemon juice and mix well.

Serve the salad fresh.
**Nutrition:**
Calories:233 Fat:2.0g
Protein:18.7g
Carbohydrates:35.5g

## 241. Salmon & Arugula Salad

**Preparation Time: 15 Minutes**
**Cooking Time: 10 minutes**
**Servings: 2**
**Ingredients:**
1/4 cup red onion, sliced thinly
1 1/2 tbsp fresh lemon juice
1 1/2 tbsp olive oil
1 tbsp extra-virgin olive oil
1 tbsp red-wine vinegar
2 center cut salmon fillets (6-oz each)
2/3 cup cherry tomatoes, halved
3 cups baby arugula leaves
Pepper and salt to taste
**Directions:**
In a shallow bowl, mix pepper, salt, 1 1/2 tbsp olive oil and lemon juice. Toss in salmon fillets and rub with the marinade. Allow to marinate for at least 15 minutes.

Grease a baking sheet and preheat oven to 350oF.

Bake marinated salmon fillet for 10 to 12 minutes or until flaky with skin side touching the baking sheet.

Meanwhile, in a salad bowl mix onion, tomatoes and arugula.

Season with pepper and salt. Drizzle with vinegar and oil. Toss to combine and serve right away with baked salmon on the side.
**Nutrition:**
Calories: 400
Protein: 36.6g
Carbs: 5.8g
Fat: 25.6g

## 242. Keto Bbq Chicken Pizza Soup

**Preparation Time:** 15 Minutes
**Cooking Time:** 1 Hour 10 minutes
**Servings:** 2
**Ingredients:**
6 chicken legs
1 medium red onion, diced
4 garlic cloves
1 large tomato, unsweetened
4 cups green beans
3/4 cup BBQ Sauce
11/2 cups mozzarella cheese, shredded
1/4 cup ghee
2 quarts water
2 quarts chicken stock
Salt and black pepper, to taste
Fresh cilantro, for garnishing
**Directions:**
Put chicken, water and salt in a large pot and bring to a boil.
Reduce the heat to medium-low and cook for about 75 minutes.
Shred the meat off the bones using a fork and keep aside.
Put ghee, red onions and garlic in a large soup and cook over a medium heat.
Add chicken stock and bring to a boil over a high heat.
Add green beans and tomato to the pot and cook for about 15 minutes.
AddBBQ Sauce, shredded chicken, salt and black pepper to the pot.
Ladle the soup into serving bowls and top with shredded mozzarella cheese and cilantro to serve.
**Nutrition:**
Calories: 449
Carbs: 7.1g
Fats: 32.5g
Proteins: 30.8g
Sodium: 252mg
Sugar: 4.7g

## 243. Mediterranean Garden Salad

**Preparation Time:** 15 Minutes
**Cooking Time:** 10 minutes
**Servings:** 2
**Ingredients:**
6 cups mixed greens
2 cups cherry tomatoes, halved
1 medium red onion, sliced (1/2 cup)
3 tb. Tahini paste
3 tb. Fresh lemon juice
3 tb. Balsamic vinegar
3 tb. Plus 1 tsp. Extra-virgin olive oil
3 tb. Water
1/2 tsp. salt
1/2 tsp. fresh ground black pepper
1/2 cup pine nuts
**Directions:**
In a large bowl, add mixed greens, cherry tomatoes, and red onion.
In a small bowl, whisk together tahini paste, lemon juice, balsamic vinegar, 3 tablespoons extra-virgin olive oil, water, salt, and black pepper.
Preheat a small skillet over medium-low heat for 1 minute. Add remaining 1 teaspoon extra-virgin olive oil and pine nuts, and cook, stirring to toast evenly on all sides, for 4 minutes. Transfer pine nuts to a plate, and let cool for 2 minutes.
Pour dressing over vegetables, and toss to coat evenly. Top with toasted pine nuts, and serve immediately.
**Nutrition:**
Calories 69
Fat 6.5 g
Fiber 2.6 g
Carbs 10.6 g
Protein 9.4 g

## 244. Buttery Millet
**Preparation Time:** 15 Minutes
**Cooking Time:** 10 minutes
**Servings:** 2
**Ingredients:**
1/4 cup mushrooms, sliced

3/4 cup onion, diced
1 tablespoon olive oil
1 teaspoon salt
3 tablespoons milk
1/2 cup millet
1 cup of water
1 teaspoon butter

**Directions:**

Pour olive oil in the skillet and add the onion.

Add mushrooms and roast the vegetables for 10 minutes over the medium heat. Stir them from time to time.

Meanwhile, pour water in the pan.

Add millet and salt.

Cook the millet with the closed lid for 15 minutes over the medium heat.

Then add the cooked mushroom mixture in the millet.

Add milk and butter. Mix up the millet well.

**Nutrition:**

calories 198
fat 7.7
fiber 3.5
carbs 27.9
protein 4.7

## 245. Delicata Squash Soup

**Preparation Time: 15 Minutes**
**Cooking Time: 30 minutes**
**Servings: 2**
**Ingredients:**
11/2 cups beef bone broth
1small onion, peeled and grated.
1/2 teaspoon sea salt
1/4 teaspoon poultry seasoning
2small Delicata Squash, chopped
2 garlic cloves, minced
2tablespoons olive oil
1/4 teaspoon black pepper
1 small lemon, juiced
5 tablespoons sour cream
**Directions:**

Put Delicata Squash and water in a medium pan and bring to a boil.

Reduce the heat and cook for about 20 minutes.

Drain and set aside.

Put olive oil, onions, garlic and poultry seasoning in a small sauce pan.

Cook for about 2 minutes and add broth.

Allow it to simmer for 5 minutes and remove from heat.

Whisk in the lemon juice and transfer the mixture in a blender.

Pulse until smooth and top with sour cream.

**Nutrition:**
Calories: 109
Carbs: 4.9g
Fats: 8.5g
Proteins: 3g
Sodium: 279mg
Sugar: 2.4g

## 246. Parsley Couscous And Cherries Salad

**Preparation Time: 15 Minutes**
**Cooking Time: 0 minutes**
**Servings: 2**
**Ingredients:**
2 cups hot water
1 cup couscous
1/2 cup walnuts, roasted and chopped
1/2 cup cherries, pitted
1/2 cup parsley, chopped
A pinch of sea salt and black pepper
1 tablespoon lime juice
2 tablespoons olive oil
**Directions:**

Put the couscous in a bowl, add the hot water, cover, leave aside for 10 minutes, fluff with a fork and transfer to a bowl.

Add the rest of the ingredients, toss and serve.

**Nutrition:**

calories 200
fat 6.71
fiber 7.3
carbs 8.5
protein 5

## 247. Mint Quinoa

**Preparation Time: 15 Minutes**
**Cooking Time: 10 minutes**
**Servings: 2**
**Ingredients:**

1 cup quinoa
1 1/4 cup water
4 teaspoons lemon juice
1/4 teaspoon garlic clove, diced
5 tablespoons sesame oil
2 cucumbers, chopped
1/3 teaspoon ground black pepper
1/3 cup tomatoes, chopped
1/2 oz scallions, chopped
1/4 teaspoon fresh mint, chopped

**Directions:**

Pour water in the pan. Add quinoa and boil it for 10 minutes.

Then close the lid and let it rest for 5 minutes more.

Meanwhile, in the mixing bowl mix up together lemon juice, diced garlic, sesame oil, cucumbers, ground black pepper, tomatoes, scallions, and fresh mint.

Then add cooked quinoa and carefully mix the side dish with the help of the spoon.

Store tabbouleh up to 2 days in the fridge.

**Nutrition:**

calories 168
fat 9.9
fiber 2
carbs 16.9
protein 3.6

# CHAPTER 14:

# Dinner Recipes

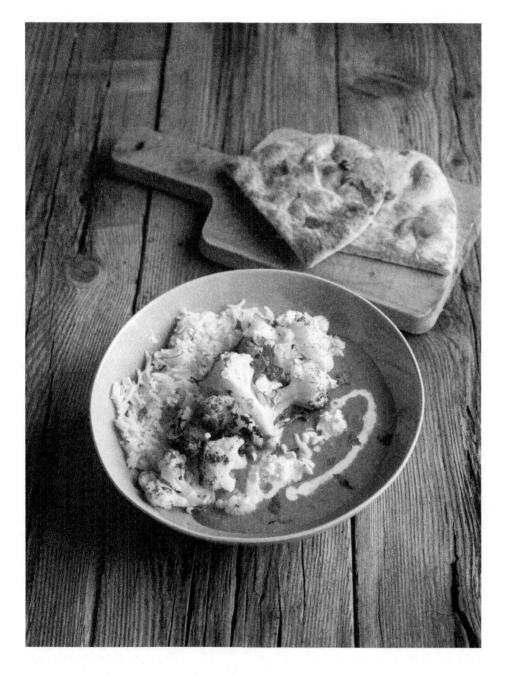

## 248. Basil Herb Salmon
**Preparation Time: 15 Minutes**
**Cooking Time:** 25 Minutes
**Servings: 3**
**Ingredients:**
1/4 Teaspoon Rosemary
2 tomato, Chopped
24 Ounces Wild Salmon
1/2 Teaspoon Oregano
1/2 Teaspoon Basil, Dried
1/4 Teaspoon Red Pepper Flakes
2 Tablespoons Balsamic Vinegar
1/4 Cup Basil, Chopped
Sea Salt & Black Pepper to Taste
2 Teaspoons Olive Oil
1 Cup Water
**Directions:**
Start by mixing your basil, pepper flakes, oregano, salt, pepper, and rosemary in a mixing bowl.

Use the mix to season your salmon, and wrap the salmon in a baking sheet, making sure it's sealed. Make sure it's a baking sheet that fits into your instant pot.

Open the lid of your instant pot and pour in your water before adding in your steamer basket. Place your salmon in the trivet, and then seal the lid. Cook on high pressure for eight to ten minutes, and then use a quick release.

Use a quick release, and then mix your basil, vinegar, tomatoes, salt, pepper and olive oil in a bowl. Mix your basil, vinegar, tomatoes, pepper, salt, and olive oil. Set it to the side and serve with the tomato mix.

**Nutrition:**
Protein: 36.5 Grams
Fat: 12.5 Grams
Carbs: 6.5 Grams
Sodium: 83 mg

## 249. Lamb Stew
**Preparation Time: 15 Minutes**
**Cooking Time:** 25 Minutes
**Servings: 3**
**Ingredients:**
1/2 Teaspoon Oregano
1/2 Teaspoon Basil
Sea Salt & Black Pepper to Taste
1/4 Cup Chicken Broth
1/2 Green Bell Pepper, Sliced
1/2 Red Bell Pepper, Sliced
1/4 Cup Parsley to Garnish, Minced
1/2 Tablespoon Olive Oil
1/2 Yellow Onion, Chopped
1/2 Tablespoon Garlic, Minced
1 lb. Lamb Shoulder, Trimmed & Cubed into 2 Inch Cubes
1 Cup Tomatoes, Fresh & Chopped
1 Tablespoon Tomato Paste, Sugar Free
1 1/2 Tablespoons Lemon Juice, Fresh
**Directions:**
Add in your onion, garlic and oil. Press sauté and cook for two minutes.

Add in all remaining ingredients except for your bell pepper and cook on high pressure for fifteen minutes.

Use a natural release for ten minutes and finish with a quick release.

Press sauté and cook your bell peppers for eight minutes. Stir often.

Garnish and serve warm.

**Nutrition:**
Calories: 252
Protein: 33.1 Grams
Fat: 10.4 Grams
Carbs: 5.3 Grams
Sodium: 142 mg

## 250. Steamed Garlic Chicken Breasts
**Preparation Time: 15 Minutes**
**Cooking Time:** 25 Minutes
**Servings: 3**
**Ingredients:**

1/4 Teaspoon Garlic Powder
1 Teaspoon Black Pepper
2 lbs. Chicken Breasts, Boneless & Skinless
1/8 Teaspoon Oregano
1/8 Teaspoon Basil
1 Tablespoon Olive Oil
1 Cup Water/Sea Salt to Taste

**Directions:**
Add your oil into your instant pot and season your chicken. Cook for three to four minutes per side.
Add in your water and then a trivet. Place your chicken on the trivet, and cook on high pressure for five minutes. Use a natural release to get rid of the steam before using a quick release. Serve warm.

**Nutrition:**
Calories: 155 Protein: 21.3 Grams
Fat: 7.2 Grams
Carbs: 0.3 Grams
Sodium: 62 mg

## 251. Chicken Cacciatore

**Preparation Time: 15 Minutes**
**Cooking Time:** 25 Minutes
**Servings: 3**
**Ingredients:**
2 Tablespoons Olive Oil
4 Chicken Thighs, Skinless
1/2 Cup Tomatoes, Crushed
1/4 Cup Red Bell Pepper, Diced
1/2 Teaspoon Oregano / 1/2 Cup Onion, Diced
1/2 Cup Green Bell Pepper, Diced/1 Bay Leaf
2 Tablespoons Parsley to Garnish
Sea Salt & Black Pepper to Taste

**Directions:**
Season your chicken with salt and pepper and press sauté.
Add oil in with your chicken, and cook until it's golden brown.

Add more oil and add in your onions and bell pepper. Allow it to cook for five minutes. Throw in your bay leaf, pepper, oregano, salt and tomatoes.
Cook for twentyfive minutes on high pressure.
Use a natural pressure release and garnish with parsley. It's best served over pasta.

**Nutrition:**
Calories: 249 Protein: 20.1 Grams
Fat: 17.2 Grams
Carbs: 6.6 Grams Sodium: 86 mg

## 252. Spicy Salmon

**Preparation Time: 15 Minutes**
**Cooking Time:** 25 Minutes
**Servings: 3**
**Ingredients:**
2 Tablespoons Red Chili Powder
8 Lemon Slices
2 Teaspoons Powdered Stevia
2 Cloves Garlic, Minced
2 Cups Water
2 Teaspoons Cumin, Ground
Sea Salt & Black Pepper to Taste
2 lb. Salmon Fillets, Cut into 8 Pieces

**Directions:**
Add two cups of water into your instant pot and place in your trive.t
In a different bowl add all of your ingredients except for your lemon slices make sure to mix well.
Pour this over your salmon fillet sand rub it in before placing them in your trivet.
Top with lemon slices and steam for two minutes.
Use a quick release, and serve immediately.

**Nutrition:**
Calories: 159
Protein: 22.4 Grams
Fat: 7.4 Grams
Carbs: 1.5 Grams

Sodium: 109 mg

## 253. Cheesy Salmon

**Preparation Time: 15 Minutes**
**Cooking Time:** 25 Minutes
**Servings: 3**
**Ingredients:**
1 1/2 lbs. Salmon Fillets
1 1/2 Cups Water
1/4 Cup Olive Oil
1 1/2 Tablespoons Feta Cheese, Crumbled
1 1/2 Clove Garlic, Minced
1/2 Teaspoons Oregano, Dried
3 Tablespoons Lemon Juice, Fresh / Sea Salt & Black Pepper to Taste
3 Rosemary Sprigs, Fresh / 3 Lemon Slices

**Directions:**
Get out a bowl and mix your lemon juice, oregano, pepper, salt, feta cheese and garlic. Whisk well.

Add your water to the pot and add in your steamer basket.

Arrange your salmon on top, and pour the cheese mixture over them.

Put lemon and rosemary over each fillet, and then steam for three minutes.

Use a quick release and serve warm.
**Nutrition:**
Protein: 22.5 Grams
Fat: 20.3 Grams
Carbs: 1.1 Grams
Sodium: 117 mg

## 254. Steak with Vegetables

**Preparation Time: 15 Minutes**
**Cooking Time:** 25 Minutes
**Servings: 3**
**Ingredients:**
2 Tablespoons Olive Oil, Divided
4 Tablespoons Olive Oil
2 Cloves Garlic, Crushed & Minced
6 Tablespoons Yogurt, Plain
2 Tablespoons Thyme
Sea Salt & Black Pepper to Taste
1 lb. Fillet Steak
2 Onions, Sliced
4 Zucchinis, Sliced into rounds
2 Red Peppers, Sliced into Strips

**Directions:**
Start by mixing your thyme, garlic and olive oil. Pulse it together in a food processor until smooth and then add in your salt, pepper and yogurt. Blend well before placing it to the side.

Press sauté, and then add half of your olive oil. Brown your steak until it's fully cooked before removing it from the pot. Transfer it to a platter.

Add in your remaining olive oil and sauté your red peppers, zucchini and onions.

Serve your steak and vegetables with your yogurt dressing.
**Nutrition:**
Calories: 415
Protein: 39.3 Grams
Fat: 22 Grams
Carbs: 16.7 Grams
Sodium: 116 mg

## 255. Easy Pork Strips

**Preparation Time: 15 Minutes**
**Cooking Time:** 25 Minutes
**Servings: 3**
**Ingredients:**
3 Tablespoons Sweet Paprika
2 Tablespoons Oregano, Dried/1/2 Tablespoon Cumin
2 Tablespoons Olive Oil/Sea Salt & black Pepper to Taste
3 Tablespoons Garlic, Chopped
2 lbs. Pork Tenderloin, Cut into Strips
2 Cups Vegetable Stock
2 Tablespoons Olive Oil / 4 Cups Lettuce, Chopped
**Directions:**

Combine your garlic, cumin, paprika, salt, pepper and oregano together.

After slicing your pork, coat it in your seasoning mixture and allow it to marinate for a half hour.

Press sauté on your instant pot before adding in your olive oil. Brown your pork strips for ten minutes before adding in your vegetable stock.

Seal your pot, cooking on high pressure for a half hour.

Serve with chopped lettuce

**Nutrition:**
Calories: 429
Protein: 61.3 Grams
Fat: 16.2 Grams
Carbs: 8.9 Grams
Sodium: 142 mg

## 256. Garlic Pork with Zucchini

**Preparation Time: 15 Minutes**
**Cooking Time:** 25 Minutes
**Servings: 3**
**Ingredients:**
1 Lemon, Cut into Wedges with the Peel Grated
2 Sprigs Thyme, Fresh & Stemmed
2 Tablespoons Olive Oil, Divided
1 Tablespoon Garlic, Minced
Sea Salt & Black Pepper to Taste
2 lb. Pork Loin, Sliced into Strips
1 Onion, Quartered
1 Red Pepper, Diced
1 Zucchini, Sliced into Strips
**Directions:**
Ge tout a bowl and combine your lemon zest, half of your olive oil, garlic, salt, pepper and thyme.

Mix well and marinate your pork strips in the mixture for about a half hour.

Press sauté on your instant pot, adding in your remaining oil.

Brown your pork in your instant pot for ten minutes, and then take it out and set it to the side.

Add in your red peppers, onions and zucchini, cooking until it turns soft.

Put your pork back in the pot and cook for two more minutes. Make sure that you stir frequently so that it doesn't burn and serve warm.

**Nutrition:**
Calories: 640
Protein: 63.3 Grams
Fat: 38.8 Grams
Carbs: 7.2 Grams
Sodium: 135 mg

## 257. Salmon with Tahini

**Preparation Time: 15 Minutes**
**Cooking Time:** 25 Minutes
**Servings: 3**
**Ingredients:**
1 lb. Salmon Fillets
2 Lemon Slices
2 Sprigs Rosemary, Fresh
3 Tablespoons Tahini Sauce
**Directions:**
Start by adding water into your instant pot before placing in your steamer basket.

Put your salmon in the steamer basket, and season with salt and pepper. Place your lemon and rosemary on top, and then cook on high pressure for three minutes.

Use a quick release, and drizzle with tahini sauce before serving.

**Nutrition:**
Calories: 306
Protein: 44.1 Grams
Fat: 14.2 Grams
Carbs: 1.4 Grams
Sodium: 101 mg

## 258. Mediterranean Chicken

**Preparation Time: 15 Minutes**

**Cooking Time:** 25 Minutes
**Servings: 3**
**Ingredients:**
2 lbs. Chicken Breast fillet, Sliced
1/4 Cup White Wine Mixed with 3 Tablespoons Red Wine
1 1/2 Teaspoons Oregano, Dried
2 Tablespoons Light Brown Sugar
6 Cloves Garlic, Chopped
**Directions:**
Start by pouring your wine into your instant pot, and then add in your remaining ingredients. Make sure to stir well.

Toss your chicken in, making sure it's evenly coated.

Seal the pot and cook on high pressure for ten minutes.

Use a natural pressure release before serving warm.

**Nutrition:**
Calories: 304 Protein: 44 Grams
Fat: 11.3 Grams Carbs: 4.2 Grams
Sodium: 131 mg

## 259. Mediterranean Wings
**Preparation Time: 15 Minutes**
**Cooking Time:** 25 Minutes
**Servings: 3**
**Ingredients:**
1/2 Tablespoon Oregano
1 Tablespoon Basil
1/2 Tablespoon Tarragon
8 Chicken Wings
1 Tablespoon Coconut Oil
1 Tablespoon Garlic Puree
1 Tablespoon Chicken Seasoning
**Directions:**
Start by mixing your garlic puree and herbs together.

Marinate your chicken in the mixture for one hour.

Add in your coconut oil and press sauté. Cook your chicken until it's browned on both sides, and then

remove it. Set your chicken to the side. Add in a cup of water before placing your steamer basket in.

Place your chicken in the steamer basket, and seal the pot. Cook on high pressure for ten minutes. Use a natural pressure release and serve warm.

**Nutrition:**
Calories: 280 Protein: 42.2 Grams
Fat: 11.2 Grams Carbs: 0 Grams
Sodium: 135 mg

## 260. Mediterranean Cod
**Preparation Time: 15 Minutes**
**Cooking Time: 25 Minutes**
**Servings: 3**
**Ingredients:**
6 Cod Fillets
1 Onion, Sliced
2 Tablespoons Olive Oil
1 Teaspoon Oregano
1 Tablespoon Lemon Juice, Fresh
28 Ounces Tomatoes, Canned & Diced
**Directions:**
Start by seasoning your fish fillets with salt and pepper.

Place your olive oil into the instant pot and then press sauté.

Add your cod in, cooking for three minutes per side.

Add in your remaining ingredients before mixing well and sealing your pot.

Cook on high pressure for five minutes.

Use a quick release, and pour your sauce over the cod before serving.

**Nutrition:**
Calories: 123
Protein: 21.4 Grams
Fat: 1.3 grams
Carbs: 7.1 Grams
Sodium: 78 mg

## 261. Cauliflower Risotto
**Preparation Time: 15 Minutes**
**Cooking Time:** 25 Minutes
**Servings: 3**
**Ingredients:**
2 Tablespoons Olive Oil
2 Onions, Large & Diced
1 Cup Parmesan Cheese, Grated & Divided
6 Tablespoons Olive Oil, Divided
Sea Salt & Black Pepper to Taste
2 Small Heads Cauliflower, Chunked /
4 Cloves Garlic, Minced
4 Cups Pearl Barley / 6 Cups Vegetable Broth
2 Tablespoons Butter / 4 Sprigs Thyme, Fresh
4 Tablespoons Parsley, Fresh & Chopped to Garnish

**Directions:**
Add your oil, garlic and onion and press sauté. Cook for three minutes, and then stir in your cauliflower. Cook for five more minutes.
Add all remaining ingredients except for your cheese and butter.
Cook for twentyfive minutes on high pressure.
Allow for a natural pressure release, and then stir in your cheese and butter. Serve warm.

**Nutrition:**
Calories: 372
Protein: 8.4 Grams
Fat: 18.8 Grams
Carbs: 48.2 Grams
Sodium: 69 mg

## 262. Turkey with Tomatoes
**Preparation Time: 15 Minutes**
**Cooking Time:** 25 Minutes
**Servings: 3**
**Ingredients:**
1 Tablespoon Olive oil
4 Turkey Breast Filets

1/4 Cup Basil, Fresh & Chopped
1 1/2 Cups Cherry Tomatoes, Halved
1/4 Cup Olive Tapenade

**Directions:**
Start by seasoning your turkey with salt, and then add your olive oil to your instant pot. Set it to sauté, and cook until browned on both sides.
Stir in your remaining ingredients, and cook for three minutes while siring frequently. Make sure your turkey is cooked all the way through. It's best served with a green salad.

**Nutrition:**
Calories: 188
Protein: 33.2 Grams
Fat: 5.1 Grams
Carbs: 2.8 Grams
Sodium: 3 mg

## 263. Lean Turkey Paprikash
**Preparation Time: 15 Minutes**
**Cooking Time:** 25 Minutes
**Servings: 3**
**Ingredients:**
Salt and black chili pepper, to taste
8 oz. egg noodles
2 extra virgin olive oil spoons
6 ounces of fat, sliced mushroom
1 spoonful of finely chopped onion
Lean ground turkey, 1 pound
1/2 cup of water
1 cubed chicken broth, crumbled
1 spoonful of sweet paprika
2/3 cup 2% Greek yogurt

**Directions:**
Pick up a big pot of lightly salted water over high heat to a boil. Cook pasta and drain according to package instructions.
Warmup oil over medium heat in a large skillet, then stir in mushrooms and onion, and cook until tender and lightly brown for a few minutes.

Attach turkey to pan, stirring from time to time. Stir in water and bouillon cube until the turkey is fully cooked. Stirring to mix, season with paprika, salt, and pepper.

Remove from the heat bath. Stir in yogurt and serve turkey over pasta right away.

**Nutrition:**
Calories: 456
Carbs: 45g
Fat: 14g
Protein: 35g

### 264. Pollo Fajitas

**Preparation Time: 15 Minutes**
**Cooking Time:** 25 Minutes
**Servings: 3**
**Ingredients:**
1 spoonful of Worcestershire sauce
1 spoonful of apple cider vinegar
1 tablespoon soy sauce with less sodium
1 tablespoon of chili powder
1 garlic clove, peeled and chopped
Dash hot sauce
4 (6ounce) fat trimmed, skinless chicken breasts sliced into strips
1 tablespoon of vegetable oil
1 big, thinly sliced onion
1 green chili pepper, seeded and sliced
Salt and ground black chili pepper.
8 (6inch) wholewheat tortillas
1/2 lemon juice

**Directions:**
Add Worcestershire sauce, vinegar, soy sauce, chili powder, garlic, and hot sauce in a big Ziploc container.
Attach strips of chicken to a Ziploc container. Seal tightly and cover with a shake. Let the chicken marinate within 30 minutes at room temperature (or cool down for many hours), shaking them periodically.
Warm oil over high heat in a large skillet, then put strips of chicken and marinade to the saucepan; sauté for 5 to 6 minutes.
Add onion plus green pepper to the pan, season with salt and pepper, and sauté until the chicken is thoroughly cooked, within 3 to 4 minutes further.
Hot tortillas in a microwave or nonstick pan. Cover tortillas with fajita mixture, and before serving, squeeze with lemon juice.

**Nutrition:**
Calories: 210
Carbs: 6g
Fat: 8g
Protein: 28g

### 265. Chunky Chicken Quesadilla

**Preparation Time: 15 Minutes**
**Cooking Time:** 25 Minutes
**Servings: 3**
**Ingredients:**
1 (6ounce) boneless, skinless breast of chicken, trimmed in fat
1 tablespoon lowfat sour cream
(8inch) tortillas with wholewheat
1/3 cup salsa
1 cup of chopped lettuce
1/3 cup shredded cheese with lowfat cheddar

**Directions:**
Cover a medium nonstick skillet over medium heat with cooking spray and warm. Add the chicken and cook each side for 3 to 5 minutes. Move chicken to a cutting board, once fully cooked.
Pour sour cream over 1 tortilla. Slice the chicken breast over sour cream and cover with salsa and lettuce. Sprinkle with cheese, then top with a tortilla.
Recoat skillet over low heat with cooking spray and cover—Cook quesadilla, about 3 minutes per side until golden, using a large spatula to flip it. Remove, slice, and serve from skillet.

**Nutrition:**
Calories: 190
Carbs: 23g

Fat: 7g
Protein: 9g

## 266. Chicken Fettuccine with Shiitake Mushrooms

**Preparation Time: 15 Minutes**
**Cooking Time:** 25 Minutes
**Servings: 3**
**Ingredients:**
Salt and black chili pepper, to taste
8ounce wholewheat fettuccine
2 spoonful of extra virgin olive oil
6ounce boneless, skinless breasts of chicken, trimmed with fat and cut into strips
Roasted garlic cloves and hazelnuts
2 ounces of shiitake mushrooms stemmed and sliced (about 1 to 1 1/2cups)
2 teaspoons lemon zest
2 lemon juice teaspoons
1/2 cup Parmesan grated cheese
1/2 tablespoon of fresh basil
**Directions:**
Pick up a big pot of lightly salted water over high heat to a boil. Cook fettuccine as instructed on the box. Drain the sauce, reserving 1/2 cup of water for the sauce.
In the meantime, warm oil over medium heat in a big, nonstick skillet. Attach strips of chicken, then sauté for 3 to 4 minutes.
Add mushrooms and garlic. Cook, stirring periodically, for 4 to 5 minutes until the mushrooms are tender. Add lemon zest, lemon juice, salt, and pepper to taste.
Add pasta, reserved broth, Parmesan, and basil into the skillet. Nice toss and serve.
**Nutrition:**
Calories: 444
Carbs: 43g
Fat: 13g

Protein: 33g

## 267. Chicken Yakitori

**Preparation Time: 15 Minutes**
**Cooking Time:** 25 Minutes
**Servings: 3**
**Ingredients:**
1/2 cup of soy sauce with less sodium
1/2 cup sherry or white wine to prepare
1/2 cup lowsodium chicken broth
1/2 teaspoon ginger
Pinch of garlic powder
1/2 cup scallions hacked
4 (6ounce) boneless, skinless, fatfree chicken breasts, sliced into 2inch cubes
**Directions:**
When using skewers of bamboo or metal spindles, soak in water for 30 minutes to stop burning the fuel.
Put soy sauce, sherry, chicken broth, ginger, garlic powder, and scallions into a small pot. Bring fixings to a boil over mediumhigh heat, and remove from heat immediately.
Preheat the broiler for the oven. Begin threading chicken on skewers. Coat a broiler pan using a cooking spray and placed skewers of chicken on the pan. Brush with sherry sauce to every skewer.
Place the saucepan under the broiler until the chicken is browned, 3 minutes. Remove the pan from the oven and turn over each chicken skewer, brushing the chicken sauce repeatedly.
Return the saucepan to the broiler until the chicken is well browned and cooked through. Serve.
**Nutrition:**
Calories: 160  Carbs: 8g
Fat: 7g  Protein: 16g

## 268. Muscle Meatballs

**Preparation Time: 15 Minutes**
**Cooking Time:** 25 Minutes
**Servings: 3**
**Ingredients:**
1 1/2 pound 93 percent ground turkey
2 egg whites or 6 spoonful of liquid egg white replace
1/2 cup rubbed wheat germ
1/4 cup fastcooking oats:
1 tablespoon of whole flaxseeds
1 tablespoon Parmesan cheese
1/2 teaspoon seasoning for alluse
1/4 teaspoon black chili pepper
**Directions:**
Preheat the oven to 400°F. Cover a baking dish of 9" by 13" with cooking spray. Put all the fixings in a large bowl, and mix gently together to combine.
Shape the mixture into 16 meatballs and put it in the baking platter. Bake for 7 minutes, then flip each meatball with a spatula.
Return to the oven and cook for around 8 to 13 minutes, until the meatballs are no longer pink in the middle. Serve.
**Nutrition:**
Calories: 266
Carbs: 11g
Fat: 5g
Protein: 46g

## 269. Orange and HoneyGlazed Chicken
**Preparation Time: 15 Minutes**
**Cooking Time:** 25 Minutes
**Servings: 3**
**Ingredients:**
4 (6ounce) boneless, skinless breasts of chicken trimmed in fat
2 tablespoons of orange juice
2 tablespoons of honey
1 tablespoon of lemon juice.
1/8 tablespoon salt
**Directions:**
Preheat to 375°F on the burner. Cover with cooking spray a 9inch by 13inch baking dish, and add chicken.
Combine orange juice, sugar, lemon juice, and salt in a small bowl. Baste the orange juice mixture on every piece of chicken.
Put foil over the dish and bake for 10 minutes. Remove the chicken foil, and turn it. Bake chicken for another ten to fifteen minutes until fried and the juices run free.
**Nutrition:**
Calories: 200
Carbs: 14g
Fat: 6g
Protein: 24g

## 270. Thai Basil Chicken
**Preparation Time: 15 Minutes**
**Cooking Time:** 25 Minutes
**Servings: 3**
**Ingredients:**
4 (6ounce) boneless, skinless breasts of chicken trimmed in fat
3 garlic cloves, peeled and chopped
2 jalapeño chilies, hairy
1 tablespoon fish sauce
1 tablespoon granulated sugar
1/4 cup of fresh basil
1 tablespoon fresh mint
1 spoonful of unsalted, dry roasted peanuts
**Directions:**
Break each breast into approximately 8 strips. Placed on aside. Cover a big, nonstick skillet over medium high heat with cooking spray and warm. Also, add the garlic and jalapeños. Stir continuously, stirring until garlic is only golden.
Add chicken strips and cook, frequently stirring, for about 8 to 10 minutes until chicken is thoroughly cooked. Add sugar and fish sauce,

cook for 30 seconds. Until eating, garnish with the basil, mint, and peanuts.

**Nutrition:**
Calories: 170  Carbs: 15g
Fat: 1g  Protein: 29g

## 271. Chicken Curry

**Preparation Time: 15 Minutes**
**Cooking Time:** 25 Minutes
**Servings: 3**
**Ingredients:**
1 small, chopped onion
1 clove of garlic, minced and peeled
3 spoonful of curry powder
1 tablespoon of sweet paprika
1 bay leaf
1 teaspoon cinnamon
1/2 teaspoon peeled and rubbed fresh ginger
Salt and black ground pepper to taste
4 (6ounce) boneless, skinless, fatcut chicken breasts, cut into 1inch cubes
1 tablespoon of tomato paste
1/2 cup of water
1/2 citrus
1/2 teaspoon chili Indian powder
1 cup 2% Greek yogurt
**Directions:**
Cover a large skillet over medium heat with cooking spray and hold. Sauté the onion for about 5 minutes, until translucent.
Add garlic, curry powder, paprika, bay leaf, cinnamon, ginger, salt, and pepper into the skillet; stir for 2 minutes.
Add the chicken and the tomato paste and water to the saucepan; whisk to mix. Bring liquid to a boil, lower heat to low, and cook for 10 minutes.
Stir in chili powder and lemon juice. Simmer within 5 minutes until the chicken is cooked through. Take off the heat and take off the bay leaf and remove it. Add yogurt and serve.

**Nutrition:**
Calories: 306
Carbs: 50g
Fat: 5g
Protein: 16g

## 272. Chicken and Broccoli StirFry

**Preparation Time: 15 Minutes**
**Cooking Time:** 25 Minutes
**Servings: 3**
**Ingredients:**
2 tablespoons of red wine
1 tablespoon soy sauce with less sodium
1/2 tablespoon of cornstarch
1 tablespoon of granulated sugar
1 tsp salt
Broccoli
1 red bell pepper, chopped and seeded
1/2 sliced onion
4 (6ounce) boneless, skinless, fatfree chicken breasts, trimmed into thin stripes
**Directions:**
Combine the red wine, soy sauce, cornstarch, sugar, and salt in a small cup. Whisk well with a fork until cornstarch dissolves.
Cover a big, nonstick skillet over mediumhigh heat with cooking spray and warm. Stir in broccoli, pepper bell, and onion until tender. Add chicken and stirfry for around 2 to 3 minutes until browned.
Pour soy sauce mixture over vegetables and chicken. Stirfry until sauce thickens, within 2 to 4 minutes. Take off heat and serve.

**Nutrition:**
Calories: 377
Carbs: 10g
Fat: 13g
Protein: 17g

## Greek Pita Pizza

**Preparation Time: 15 Minutes**
**Cooking Time:** 25 Minutes
**Servings: 3**
**Ingredients:**
1 (6ounce) boneless, skinless breast of chicken, trimmed in fat
Wholewheat pita bread
1/2 tablespoon extravirgin olive oil
2 Sliced olives
1 tsp vinegar with red wine
1/2 clove of garlic, minced and peeled
1/4 teaspoon of dried oregano
1/4 teaspoon of dried basil
Salt and black chili pepper, to taste
1/4 cup fresh spinach
Lowfat cheese crumbled
1/2 tomatoes, seeded, chopped

**Directions:**
Preheat the broiler to high on the burner. Cover a small skillet over medium heat with cooking spray and hold. Put the chicken in the skillet and cook for 3 to 5 minutes.

When juices run clear, remove chicken from the heat; set aside. Let the chicken breast cool, and then chop into small bits.

In the meantime, put pita bread on a baking sheet, and brush with oil lightly. Broil up for 2 minutes 4 inches from the sun.

Put olives, vinegar, garlic, oregano, basil, salt, chili pepper, and any remaining oil in a small cup. Healthy balance to blend.

Layer a mixture of olives over the pita. Then put the spinach, feta, onion, and chicken. Broil until the feta gets warm and softened, about 3 minutes more.

**Nutrition:**
Calories: 200
Carbs: 33g
Fat: 5g

Protein: 6g

## 273. BowTie Pasta Salad with Chicken and Chickpeas

**Preparation Time: 15 Minutes**
**Cooking Time:** 25 Minutes
**Servings: 3**
**Ingredients:**
Salt, just to taste
Wholewheat bowtie pasta 8 ounces
3 (6ounce) fatcut chicken breasts, fried, shredded
1/2 (15 ounces) of chickpeas can be drained and rinsed
1 canned sliced black olive (2.25ounce), drained
Celery stalks, shredded
2 cucumbers, split
1/2 cup shredded carrots
1/2 yellow, finely chopped onion
Sliced Parmesan cheese
1 tbsp of extra virgin olive oil
1/3 cup red vinegar
1/2 teaspoon Worcestershire sauce
1/2 tablespoon of spicy brown mustard
1/2 clove of garlic, minced and peeled
1 tbsp basil chopped or 1 teaspoon dried basil
1/4 teaspoon black chili pepper

**Directions:**
Pick up a big pot of lightly salted water over high heat to a boil. Cook the pasta, as stated in the instructions box. Drain and run the pasta for about 30 seconds under cold water, or until it is fully cool.

Move pasta to a big bowl and add the ingredients leftover. To blend, use tongs to mix thoroughly. Cover the bowl and cool for at least 1/2 hours or till night. Throw in the salad before serving.

**Nutrition:**

Calories: 317
Carbs: 44g
Fat: 12g
Protein: 8g

## 274. Greek Style Quesadillas
**Preparation Time: 15 Minutes**
**Cooking Time:** 25 Minutes
**Servings: 3**
Ingredients:
4 wholewheat tortillas
1 cup Mozzarella cheese, shredded
1 cup fresh spinach, chopped
2 tablespoon Greek yogurt
1 egg, beaten
1/4 cup green olives, sliced
1 tablespoon olive oil
1/3 cup fresh cilantro, chopped
**Directions:**
In the bowl, combine mozzarella cheese, spinach, yogurt, egg, olives, and cilantro. Then pour olive oil into the skillet.
In the skillet, place one tortilla and spread it with a mozzarella mixture. Top it with the second tortilla and spread it with cheese mixture again.
Then place the third tortilla and spread it with all remaining cheese mixture. Cover it with the last tortilla and fry it for 5 minutes from each side over medium heat.
**Nutrition:**
Calories: 193
Fat: 7.7g
Carbs: 23.6g
Protein: 8.3g

## 275. Light Paprika Moussaka
**Preparation Time: 15 Minutes**
**Cooking Time:** 25 Minutes
**Servings: 3**
Ingredients:
1 eggplant, trimmed
1 cup ground chicken

1/3 cup white onion, diced
3 oz. Cheddar cheese, shredded
1 potato, sliced
1 teaspoon olive oil
1 teaspoon salt
1/2 cup milk
1 tablespoon butter
1 tablespoon ground paprika
1 tablespoon Italian seasoning
1 teaspoon tomato paste
**Directions:**
Slice the eggplant in length and sprinkle with salt. In the skillet, pour olive oil and add sliced potato. Roast potato for 2 minutes from each side. Then transfer it to the plate.
Put eggplant in the skillet and roast it for 2 minutes from each side too. In the pan, pour milk and bring it to a boil, then put the tomato paste, Italian seasoning, paprika, butter, and cheddar cheese.
Then mix up together onion with ground chicken. Arrange the sliced potato in the casserole in one layer. Then add 1/2 part of all sliced eggplants.
Spread the eggplants with 1/2 part of the chicken mixture. Then add the remaining eggplants. Pour the milk mixture over the eggplants—Bake moussaka for 30 minutes at 355F. Serve.
**Nutrition:**
Calories: 387
Fat: 21.2g
Carbs: 26.3g
Protein: 25.4g

## 276. Cucumber Bowl with Spices and Greek Yogurt
**Preparation Time: 15 Minutes**
**Cooking Time:** 25 Minutes
**Servings: 3**
Ingredients:

4 cucumbers
1/2 teaspoon chili pepper
1/4 cup fresh parsley, chopped
3/4 cup fresh dill, chopped
2 tablespoons lemon juice
1/2 teaspoon salt
1/2 teaspoon ground black pepper
1/4 teaspoon sage
1/2 teaspoon dried oregano
1/3 cup Greek yogurt

**Directions:**

Make the cucumber dressing: blend the dill and parsley until you get green mash. Then combine green mash with lemon juice, salt, ground black pepper, sage, dried oregano, Greek yogurt, and chili pepper. Churn the mixture well.

Chop the cucumbers roughly and combine them with cucumber dressing. Mix up well. Refrigerate the cucumber for 20 minutes. Serve.

**Nutrition:**
Calories: 114
Fat: 1.6g
Carbs: 23.2g
Protein: 7.6g

## 277. Sweet Potato Bacon Mash

**Preparation Time: 15 Minutes**
**Cooking Time:** 25 Minutes
**Servings: 3**
**Ingredients:**
3 sweet potatoes, peeled
4 oz. bacon, chopped
1 cup chicken stock
1 tablespoon butter
1 teaspoon salt
2 oz. Parmesan, grated

**Directions:**

Dice sweet potato and put it in the pan. Add chicken stock and close the lid. Boil the vegetables until they are soft. After this, drain the chicken stock.

Mash the sweet potato with the help of the potato masher. Add grated cheese and butter. Mix up together salt and chopped bacon. Fry the mixture until it is crunchy (1015 minutes).

Add cooked bacon to the mashed sweet potato and mix up with the help of the spoon. It is recommended to serve the meal warm or hot.

**Nutrition:**
Calories: 304
Fat: 18.1
Carbs: 18.8
Protein: 17

## 278. Prosciutto Wrapped Mozzarella Balls

**Preparation Time: 15 Minutes**
**Cooking Time:** 25 Minutes
**Servings: 3**
**Ingredients:**
8 Mozzarella balls, cherry size
4 oz. bacon, sliced
1/4 teaspoon ground black pepper
3/4 teaspoon dried rosemary
1 teaspoon butter

**Directions:**

Sprinkle the sliced bacon with ground black pepper and dried rosemary. Wrap every mozzarella ball in the sliced bacon and secure them with toothpicks. Melt butter.

Brush wrapped mozzarella balls with butter. Line the baking tray with the parchment and arrange mozzarella balls in it. Bake the meal for 10 minutes at 365F. Serve.

**Nutrition:**
Calories: 323
Fat: 26.8 g
Carbs: 0.6 g
Protein: 20.6 g

## 279. Chicken and Cabbage Mix

**Preparation Time: 15 Minutes**
**Cooking Time:** 25 Minutes
**Servings: 3**
**Ingredients:**
3 medium chicken breasts, skinless, boneless and cut into thin strips
4 ounces green cabbage, shredded
5 tablespoon extravirgin olive oil
Salt and black pepper to taste
2 tablespoons sherry vinegar
tablespoon chives, chopped
1/4 cup feta cheese, crumbled
1/4 cup barbeque sauce
bacon slices, cooked and crumbled
**Directions:**
In a bowl, mix 4 tablespoon oil with vinegar, salt and pepper to taste and stir well.
Add the shredded cabbage, toss to coat and leave aside for now.
Season chicken with salt and pepper, heat a pan with remaining oil over medium high heat, add chicken, cook for 6 minutes, take off heat, transfer to a bowl and mix well with barbeque sauce.
Arrange salad on serving plates, add chicken strips, sprinkle cheese, chives and crumbled bacon and serve right away.
**Nutrition:**
Calories:200,
Fat:15g,
Fiber:3g,
Carbs:10g,
Protein:33g

## 280. Green Onion, Rice With Shrimps

**Preparation Time: 15 Minutes**
**Cooking Time:** 25 Minutes
**Servings: 3**
**Ingredients:**
2 Cups White Rice
7 Oz Boiled Shrimps

2 Tablespoon Olive Oil
2 Eggs
1 Cup Frozen Peas
1 Green Onion
2 Garlic Cloves
2 Tablespoon Rice Vinegar
3 Tablespoon Soy Sauce
1 Teaspoon Ground Ginger
1/2 Teaspoon Ground Allspice
A Pinch Of Salt
**Directions:**
Heat Deep Frying Pan; Add 1 Tablespoon Oil. Season Shrimps With Salt And Pepper.
Fry For 3 Minutes And Place On A Plate.
Add Oil And Fry Chopped Green Onion, Garlic And Ginger Powder. Fry For 2 Minutes.
Add Washed Rice Into The Frying Pan, Stir And Simmer For 2 Minutes.
Add The Eggs, Stir And Fry For Another 2 Minutes. Add Peas, Vinegar, Soy Sauce, 1/2 Cup Of Water And Simmer Until Rice Is Ready.
Add Shrimps And Steam Again For 3 Minutes. Sprinkle Rice With Green Onion.
**Nutrition:**
Calories:342, Fat:3g,
Fiber:3g, Carbs:5g, Protein:4g

## 281. Portobello & Wine Stew

**Preparation Time: 15 Minutes**
**Cooking Time:** 25 Minutes
**Servings: 3**
**Ingredients:**
1 Lb Portobello
5 Tomatoes
1/2 Cup Dry White Wine
1/2 Teaspoon Dry Oregano
2 Garlic Cloves
2 Tablespoon Olive Oil
A Pinch Of Salt
**Directions:**

Scald Tomatoes, Peel And Cut Into Thin Rings. Mince The Garlic.

*Preheat The Frying Pan With Oil. Add Garlic, Tomatoes And Oregano. Season Tomato Dressing With Salt, Add Wine And Simmer For 10 Minutes.

*Peel And Cut Mushrooms Into Thin Slices. Add To Other Ingredients, Stir And Stew For 10 Minutes.

**Nutrition:**
Calories:200,
Fat:15g, Fiber:3g,
Carbs:10g, Protein:33g

## 282. Pesto Sauce Zucchini Spaghetti

**Preparation Time: 15 Minutes**
**Cooking Time:** 25 Minutes
**Servings: 3**
**Ingredients:**
3 Zucchini
4 Oz Feta
6 Cherry Tomatoes
2 Wholegrain Bread Slices
2 Tablespoon Pesto Sauce
4 Tablespoon Olive Oil
A Pinch Of Ground Coriander And Salt

**Directions:**
Cover A Baking Sheet With Parchment. Cut Tomatoes Into Halves, Season With Oil, Salt And Coriander.

*Place On A Baking Sheet And Bake For 20 Minutes At 190°C (374°F). Stir 23 Times While Baking.

*Cut Bread Slices Into Small Cubes. Dry On A Dry Frying Pan.

*Wash And Cut Zucchini Into Spaghetti With A Vegetable Slicer. Heat The Frying Pan, Add Oil, Add The Zucchini And Fry For 3 Minutes.

*Place Hot Spaghetti On A Plate, Add Pesto.

*Top With Chopped Feta, Tomatoes, And Bread Croutons.

**Nutrition:**
Calories:230,
Fat:12g,
Fiber:12g,
Carbs:34g,
Protein:13g

## 283. Lemon Juice Avocado Spread

**Preparation Time: 15 Minutes**
**Cooking Time:** 25 Minutes
**Servings: 3**
**Ingredients:**
1 Ripe Avocado, Peeled And Pitted
1 Teaspoon Freshly Squeezed Lemon Juice
6 Boneless Sardine Filets (Packed In Olive Oil)
1/4 Cup Diced Sweet White Onion
1 Stalk Celery, Diced
1/2 Teaspoon Salt
1/4 Teaspoon Freshly Ground Black Pepper

**Directions:**
Combine The Avocado, Lemon Juice, And Sardine Filets In A Blender Or Food Processor, And Pulse Just Until Fairly Smooth. A Few Chunks Are Fine For Texture.

*Spoon The Mixture Into A Clean Small Bowl And Add The Onion, Celery, Salt, And Pepper.

*Mix Well With A Fork And Serve As Desired.

**Nutrition:**
Calories:145,
Fat:4g,
Fiber:3g,
Carbs:11g,
Protein:4g

## 284. Lovely Stuffed Tomatoes

**Preparation Time: 15 Minutes**
**Cooking Time:** 25 Minutes
**Servings: 3**
**Ingredients:**
4 Large, Ripe Tomatoes
1 Tablespoon Extra Virgin Olive Oil
2 Garlic Cloves, Minced
1/2 Cup Diced Yellow Onion
1/2-Pound White Or Cremini Mushrooms, Sliced
1 Tablespoon Chopped Fresh Basil
1 Tablespoon Chopped Fresh Oregano
1/2 Teaspoon Salt
1/4 Teaspoon Freshly Ground Black Pepper
1 Cup Shredded Part Skim Mozzarella Cheese
1 Tablespoon Grated Parmesan Cheese
**Directions:**
Preheat The Oven To 375°F. Line A Baking Sheet With Aluminum Foil.
Slice The Bottom Of Each Tomato So They Will Stand Upright Without Wobbling. Cut A 1/2inch Slice From The Top Of Each Tomato And Use A Spoon To Gently Remove Most Of The Pulp, Placing It In A Clean Medium Bowl. Place The Tomatoes On The Baking Sheet.
In A Medium Skillet, Heat The Olive Oil On A Medium Heat. Sauté The Mushrooms, Oregano, Garlic, Onion And Basil For 5 Minutes, And Season With Salt And Pepper.
Pour The Mixture Into A Clean Bowl And Blend With The Tomato Pulp. Stir In The Mozzarella Cheese.
Fill Each Tomato With The Mixture, Top With Parmesan Cheese, And Bake Until The Cheese Is Full Of Bubble, 15 To 20 Minutes.
Serve Immediately.
**Nutrition:**

Calories:230,
Fat:12g,
Fiber:12g,
Carbs:34g,
Protein:13g

## 285. Roasted Veggie Soup
**Preparation Time: 15 Minutes**
**Cooking Time:** 25 Minutes
**Servings: 3**
**Ingredients:**
2 Sweet Potatoes, Peeled And Sliced
2 Parsnips, Peeled And Sliced
2 Carrots, Peeled And Sliced
2 Tablespoons Extravirgin Olive Oil
1 Teaspoon Chopped Fresh Rosemary
1 Teaspoon Chopped Fresh Thyme
1 Teaspoon Salt
1/2 Teaspoon Freshly Ground Black Pepper
4 Cups Vegetable Or Chicken Broth
Grated Parmesan Cheese For Garnish (Optional)
**Directions:**
Preheat The Oven To 400°F. Line A Baking Sheet With Aluminum Foil.
Combine The Sweet Potatoes, Parsnips, And Carrots In A Large Bowl. Add The Olive Oil And Toss To Coat.
Put The Thyme, Rosemary, Salt, And Pepper, Tossing Well.
Spread The Vegetables On A Baking Sheet And Roast Until Tender, About 30 To 35 Minutes. Take Out The Baking Sheet From Oven And Allow To Cool.
Transfer Of The Vegetables And Broth To A Blender Or Food Processor (Working In Batches) And Blend Until Smooth.
Pour Each Blended Puree Batch Into A Large Saucepan And Heat The Soup Over Low Heat Until Heated Through.

Spoon Into Clean Bowls And Top With Parmesan Cheese (Optional).

**Nutrition:**
Calories: 20
Fat: 1.2g
Protein: 0.6g
Carbs: 4.4g
Fiber: 0.6g
Sodium: 12mg

## 286. Palatable Chicken Breasts

**Preparation Time: 15 Minutes**
**Cooking Time:** 25 Minutes
**Servings: 3**
**Ingredients:**
1/4 Cup Plus 1 Tablespoon Extra Virgin Olive Oil
4 Boneless, Skinless Chicken Breasts
1/2 Teaspoon Salt
1/4 Teaspoon Freshly Ground Black Pepper
1 Packed Cup Fresh Basil Leaves
1 Garlic Clove, Minced
1/4 Cup Grated Parmesan Cheese
1/4 Cup Pine Nuts
**Directions:**
Add 1 Tablespoon Of The Olive Oil To A Large Skillet And Heat On Medium High.
Season The Whole Chicken Breasts On Both Sides With Salt And Pepper And Add To The Skillet.
Cook For 10 Minutes On The First Side, Then Flip And Cook For 5 Minutes.
Meanwhile, Add The Basil, Garlic, Parmesan Cheese, And Pine Nuts To A Blender And Blend On High. Gently Pour In The Remaining 1/4 Cup Olive Oil And Blend Until Smooth.
Add 1 Tablespoon Pesto On Each Chicken Breast And Spread All Over, Cover The Skillet, And Cook For 5 Minutes.

Serve The Chicken Pesto Side Up.
**Nutrition:**
Calories: 179
Fat: 15.5g
Protein: 5.1g
Carbs: 6.8g
Fiber: 3.0g
Sodium: 324mg

## 287. Moist Shredded Beef

**Preparation Time: 15 Minutes**
**Cooking Time:** 25 Minutes
**Servings: 3**
**Ingredients:**
2 lbs beef roast beef, cut into chunks
1/2 tbsp dried red pepper
1 tbsp Italian seasoning
1 tbsp garlic, minced
2 tbsp vinegar
14 oz can fireroasted tomatoes
1/2 cup bell pepper, chopped
1/2 cup carrots, chopped
1 cup onion, chopped
1 tsp salt
**Directions:**
Add all ingredients into the inner pot of the instant pot and set the pot on sauté mode.
Seal pot with lid and cook on high for 20 minutes.
Once done, release pressure using quick release.
Remove lid.
Shred the meat using a fork.
Stir well and serve.
**Nutrition:**
Calories 456,
Fat 32.7g
Carbs 7.7g
Sugar 4.1g
Protein 31g
Cholesterol 118 mg

## 288. Braised Beef In OreganoTomato Sauce

**Preparation Time: 15 Minutes**
**Cooking Time:** 25 Minutes
**Servings: 3**
**Ingredients:**
2 onions, chopped
3 celery stalks, diced
4 cloves garlic, minced
2 (28ounce) cans of Italianstyle stewed tomatoes
1 cup dry red vine
1 teaspoon dried oregano
1 teaspoon salt
3 pounds boneless beef chuck roast, cut into 11/2 inch cubes
1/2 cup chopped fresh parsley
1/4 cup vegetable oil
3/4 teaspoon black pepper
**Directions:**
Place a pot on mediumhigh fire and heat for 2 minutes.
Add oil and heat for another 2 minutes.

Add beef and brown on all sides. Around 12 minutes.
Add onions, celery, and garlic, and sauté for 5 minutes or until vegetables are tender. Add remaining ingredients and bring to a boil.
Reduce heat to low, cover, and simmer for 60 minutes or until beef is forktender.
**Nutrition:**
Calories 285
Carbs 7.4g
Protein 31.7g
 Fat 14.6g

## 289. Pork Chops And Herbed Tomato Sauce

**Preparation Time: 15 Minutes**
**Cooking Time:** 25 Minutes
**Servings: 3**
**Ingredients:**
4 pork loin chops, boneless
6 tomatoes, peeled and crushed

3 tablespoons parsley, chopped
2 tablespoons olive oil
1/4 cup kalamata olives, pitted and halved
1 yellow onion, chopped
1 garlic clove, minced
**Directions:**
Heat up a pan with the oil over medium heat, add the pork chops, cook them for 3 minutes on each side, and divide between plates.
Heat up the same pan again over medium heat, add the tomatoes, parsley, and the rest of the ingredients, whisk, simmer for 4 minutes, drizzle over the chops and serve.
**Nutrition:**
Calories 334
Fat 17g
Fiber 2g
Carbs 12g
Protein 34g

## 290. Beef Shawarma

**Preparation Time: 15 Minutes**
**Cooking Time:** 25 Minutes
**Servings: 3**
**Ingredients:**
1/2 lb ground beef
1/4 tsp cinnamon
1/2 tsp dried oregano
1 cup cabbage, cut into strips
1/2 cup bell pepper, sliced
1/4 tsp ground coriander
1/2 tsp cumin
1/4 tsp cayenne pepper
1/4 tsp ground allspice
1/2 cup onion, chopped
1/2 tsp salt
**Directions:**
Set instant pot on sauté mode.
Add meat to the pot and sauté until brown.
Add remaining ingredients and stir well.

Seal pot with lid and cook on high for 5 minutes.

Once done, release pressure using quick release. Remove lid.

**Nutrition:**
Calories 245
Fat 7.4g
Carbs 7.9g
Sugar 3.9g
Protein 35.6g
Cholesterol 101mg

# 291. Beef Brisket And Veggies

**Preparation Time: 15 Minutes**
**Cooking Time:** 25 Minutes
**Servings: 3**
**Ingredients:**
3pound beef brisket
1 carrot, peeled, chopped
1 onion, peeled
1 garlic clove, peeled
1 teaspoon peppercorns
1 teaspoon salt
1 teaspoon ground black pepper
1/2 bay leaf
1/2 cup crushed tomatoes
3 cups of water
1 celery stalk, chopped
**Directions:**
Place the beef brisket in the saucepan.
Add carrot, onion, garlic clove, peppercorns, salt, ground black pepper, bay leaf, crushed tomatoes, celery stalk, and water.
Close the lid and bring the meat to a boil.
Simmer the meal for 4 hours over medium heat.
Serve the meat poached vegetables.
**Nutrition:**
Calories 321
Fat 10.5g
Fiber 0.9g
Carbs 3g,

Protein 50.4g

# 292. Beef Curry
**Preparation Time: 15 Minutes**
**Cooking Time:** 25 Minutes
**Servings: 3**
**Ingredients:**
1/2 lb beef stew meat, cubed
1 bell peppers, sliced
1 cup beef stock
1 tbsp fresh ginger, grated
1/2 tsp ground cumin
1 tsp ground coriander
1/2 tsp cayenne pepper
1/2 cup sunroasted tomatoes, diced
2 tbsp olive oil
1 tsp garlic, crushed
1 green chili peppers, chopped
**Directions:**
Add all ingredients into the instant pot and stir well.
Seal pot with lid and cook on high for 30 minutes.
Once done, allow to release pressure naturally. Remove lid.
Serve and enjoy.
**Nutrition:**
Calories 391
Fat 21.9g
Carbs 11.6g
Sugar 5.8g
Protein 37.4g
Cholesterol 101mg

# 293. Hearty Beef Ragu
**Preparation Time: 15 Minutes**
**Cooking Time:** 25 Minutes
**Servings: 3**
**Ingredients:**
1 1/2 lbs beef steak. Diced
1 1/2 cup beef stock
1 tbsp coconut amino
14 oz can tomatoes, chopped
1/2 tsp ground cinnamon
1 tsp dried oregano

1 tsp dried thyme
1 tsp dried basil
1 tsp paprika
1 bay leaf
1 tbsp garlic, chopped
1/2 tsp cayenne pepper
1 celery stick, diced
1 carrot, diced
1 onion, diced
2 tbsp olive oil
1/4 tsp pepper
1 1/2 tsp sea salt

**Directions:**

Add oil into the instant pot and set the pot on sauté mode.

Add celery, carrots, onion, and salt and sauté for 5 minutes.

Add meat and remaining ingredients and stir everything well.

Seal pot with lid and cook on high for 30 minutes.

Once done, allow to release pressure naturally for 10 minutes, then release remaining using quick release. Remove lid.

Shred meat using a fork. Set pot on sauté mode and cook for 10 minutes. Stir every 23 minutes.

Serve and enjoy.

**Nutrition:**
Calories 435
Fat 18.1g,
Carbs 12.3g
 Sugar 5.5g
Protein 54.4g
Cholesterol 152mg

## 294. Hot Pork Meatballs

**Preparation Time: 15 Minutes**
**Cooking Time:** 25 Minutes
**Servings: 3**
**Ingredients:**
4 oz pork loin, grinded
1/2 teaspoon garlic powder
1/4 teaspoon chili powder

1/4 teaspoon cayenne pepper
1/4 teaspoon ground black pepper
1/4 teaspoon white pepper
1 tablespoon water
1 teaspoon olive oil

**Directions:**

Mix up together garlic powder, cayenne pepper, ground black pepper, white pepper, and water.

With the help of the fingertips, make the small meatballs.

Heat up olive oil in the skillet.

Range in the oil and cook for 10 minutes totally. Flip on another side from time to time.

**Nutrition:**
Calories 162
Fat 10.3g
Fiber 0.3g
Carbs 1g
Protein 15.7g

## 295. Beef And Zucchini Skillet

**Preparation Time: 15 Minutes**
**Cooking Time:** 25 Minutes
**Servings: 3**
**Ingredients:**
2 oz ground beef
1/2 onion, sliced
1/2 bell pepper, sliced
1 tablespoon butter
1/2 teaspoon salt
1 tablespoon tomato sauce
1 small zucchini, chopped
1/2 teaspoon dried oregano

**Directions:**

Place the ground beef in the skillet.

Add salt, butter, and dried oregano.

Mix up the meat mixture and cook it for 10 minutes.

After this, transfer the cooked ground beef to the bowl.

Place zucchini, bell pepper, and onion in the skillet (where the ground meat was cooking) and roast the vegetables for 7 minutes over medium heat or until they are tender.

Then add cooked ground beef and tomato sauce. Mix up well.

Cook the beef toss for 23 minutes over medium heat.

**Nutrition:**
Calories 182
Fat 8.7g
Fiber 0.1g
Carbs 0.3g
Protein 24.1g

## 296. Meatloaf

**Preparation Time: 15 Minutes**
**Cooking Time:** 25 Minutes
**Servings: 3**
**Ingredients:**
2 lbs. ground beef
2 eggs, lightly beaten
1/4 tsp dried basil
3 tbsp olive oil
1/2 tsp dried sage
1 1/2 tsp dried parsley
1 tsp oregano
1 tsp thyme
1 tsp rosemary
Pepper
Salt

**Directions:**
Pour 1 1/2 cups of water into the instant pot, then place the trivet in the pot.

Spray loaf pan with cooking spray.

Add all ingredients into the mixing bowl and mix until well combined.

Transfer meat mixture into the prepared loaf pan and place loaf pan on top of the trivet in the pot.

Seal pot with lid and cook on high for 35 minutes.

Once done, allow to release pressure naturally for 10 minutes, then release

remaining using quick release. Remove lid.

Serve and enjoy.

**Nutrition:**
Calories 365
Fat 18g
Carbs 0.7g
Sugar 0.1g
Protein 47.8g
Cholesterol 190mg

## 297. Tasty Lamb Ribs

**Preparation Time: 15 Minutes**
**Cooking Time:** 25 Minutes
**Servings: 3**
**Ingredients:**
2 garlic cloves, minced
1/4 cup shallot, chopped
2 tablespoons fish sauce
1/2 cup veggie stock
2 tablespoons olive oil
1 and 1/2 tablespoons lemon juice
1 tablespoon coriander seeds, ground
1 tablespoon ginger, grated
Salt and black pepper to the taste
2 pounds lamb ribs

**Directions:**
In a roasting pan, combine the lamb with the garlic, shallots, and the rest of the ingredients, toss, introduce in the oven at 300 degrees F and cook for 2 hours.

Divide the lamb between plates and serve with a side salad.

**Nutrition:**
Calories 293
Fat 9.1g
Fiber 9.6g
Carbs 16.7g
Protein 2402g

## 298. Mediterranean Pork Roast

**Preparation Time: 15 Minutes**
**Cooking Time:** 25 Minutes

**Servings: 3**
**Ingredients:**
2 tablespoons Olive oil
2 pounds Pork roast
1/2 teaspoon Paprika
3/4 cup Chicken broth
2 teaspoons Dried sage
1/2 tablespoon Garlic minced
1/4 teaspoon Dried marjoram
1/4 teaspoon Dried Rosemary
1 teaspoon Oregano
1/4 teaspoon Dried thyme
1 teaspoon Basil
1/4 teaspoon Kosher salt
**Directions:**
In a small bowl mix broth, oil, salt, and spices. In a skillet pour olive oil and bring to mediumhigh heat. Put the pork into it and roast until all sides become brown.

Take out the pork after cooking and poke the roast all over with a knife. Place the poked pork roast into a 6quart crock pot. Now, pour the small bowl mixture liquid all over the roast.

Seal crock pot and cook on low for 8 hours. After cooking, remove it from the crock pot on to a cutting board and shred into pieces. Afterward, add the shredded pork back into the crockpot. Simmer it another 10 minutes. Serve along with feta cheese, pita bread, and tomatoes.

**Nutrition:**
Calories 361
Fat 10.4g
Carbohydrates 0.7g
Protein 43.8g

## 299. *Beef Pizza*
**Preparation Time: 15 Minutes**
**Cooking Time:** 25 Minutes
**Servings: 3**
**Ingredients:**
For Crust:

3 cups allpurpose flour
1 tablespoon sugar
21/4 teaspoons active dry yeast
1 teaspoon salt
2 tablespoons olive oil
1 cup warm water
 For Topping:
1pound ground beef
1 medium onion, chopped
2 tablespoons tomato paste
1 tablespoon ground cumin
Salt and ground black pepper, as required
1/4 cup water
1 cup fresh spinach, chopped
8 ounces artichoke hearts, quartered
4 ounces fresh mushrooms, sliced
2 tomatoes, chopped
4 ounces feta cheese, crumbled
**Directions:**
Mix the flour, sugar, yeast and salt with a stand mixer, using the dough hook. Add 2 tablespoons of the oil and warm water and knead until a smooth and elastic dough is formed.

Make a ball of the dough and set aside for about 15 minutes.

Situate the dough onto a lightly floured surface and roll into a circle. Situate the dough into a lightly, greased round pizza pan and gently, press to fit. Set aside for about 1015 minutes. Coat the crust with some oil. Preheat the oven to 400 degrees F.

For topping:

Fry beef in a nonstick skillet over mediumhigh heat for about 45 minutes. Mix in the onion and cook for about 5 minutes, stirring frequently. Add the tomato paste, cumin, salt, black pepper and water and stir to combine.

Put heat to medium and cook for about 510 minutes. Remove from the heat and set aside. Place the beef mixture over the pizza crust and top with the spinach, followed by the artichokes, mushrooms, tomatoes, and Feta cheese.

Bake until the cheese is melted. Pullout from the oven and keep aside for about 35 minutes before slicing. Cut into desired sized slices and serve.

**Nutrition:**
Calories 309
Fat 8.7g
Carbohydrates 3.7g
Protein 3.3g

## 300. Beef & Bulgur Meatballs

**Preparation Time: 15 Minutes**
**Cooking Time:** 25 Minutes
**Servings: 3**
**Ingredients:**
3/4 cup uncooked bulgur
1pound ground beef
1/4 cup shallots, minced
1/4 cup fresh parsley, minced
1/2 teaspoon ground allspice
1/2 teaspoon ground cumin
1/2 teaspoon ground cinnamon
1/4 teaspoon red pepper flakes, crushed
Salt, as required
1 tablespoon olive oil

**Directions:**
In a large bowl of the cold water, soak the bulgur for about 30 minutes. Drain the bulgur well and then, squeeze with your hands to remove the excess water. In a food processor, add the bulgur, beef, shallot, parsley, spices and salt and pulse until a smooth mixture is formed.

Situate the mixture into a bowl and refrigerate, covered for about 30 minutes. Remove from the refrigerator and make equal sized balls from the beef mixture. Using big nonstick skillet,

heat up the oil over mediumhigh heat and cook the meatballs in 2 batches for about 1314 minutes, flipping frequently. Serve warm

**Nutrition:**
Calories 228 Fat 7.4g
Carbohydrates 0.1g
Protein 3.5g

## 301. Balsamic Beef Dish

**Preparation Time: 15 Minutes**
**Cooking Time:** 25 Minutes
**Servings: 3**
**Ingredients:**
3 pounds chuck roast
3 cloves garlic, thinly sliced
1 tablespoon oil
1 teaspoon flavored vinegar
1/2 teaspoon pepper
1/2 teaspoon rosemary
1 tablespoon butter
1/2 teaspoon thyme
1/4 cup balsamic vinegar
1 cup beef broth

**Directions:**
Slice the slits in the roast and stuff in garlic slices all over. Combine flavored vinegar, rosemary, pepper, thyme and rub the mixture over the roast. Select the pot on sauté mode and mix in oil, allow the oil to heat up. Cook both side of the roast.

Take it out and set aside. Stir in butter, broth, balsamic vinegar and deglaze the pot. Return the roast and close the lid, then cook on HIGH pressure for 40 minutes.

Perform a quick release. Serve!

**Nutrition:**
Calories 393
Fat 15g
Carbohydrates 25g
Protein 37g

## 302. Chicken with Caper Sauce

**Preparation Time: 15 Minutes**
**Cooking Time:** 25 Minutes
**Servings: 3**
**Ingredients:**
For Chicken:
2 eggs
Salt and ground black pepper, as required
1 cup dry breadcrumbs
2 tablespoons olive oil
11/2 pounds skinless, boneless chicken breast halves, pounded into 3/4inch thickness and cut into pieces
 For Capers Sauce:
3 tablespoons capers
1/2 cup dry white wine
3 tablespoons fresh lemon juice
Salt and ground black pepper, as required
2 tablespoons fresh parsley, chopped
**Directions:**
For chicken: in a shallow dish, add the eggs, salt and black pepper and beat until well combined. In another shallow dish, place breadcrumbs. Soak the chicken pieces in egg mixture then coat with the breadcrumbs evenly. Shake off the excess breadcrumbs.
Cook the oil over medium heat and cook the chicken pieces for about 57 minutes per side or until desired doneness. With a slotted spoon, situate the chicken pieces onto a paper towel lined plate. With a piece of the foil, cover the chicken pieces to keep them warm.
In the same skillet, incorporate all the sauce ingredients except parsley and cook for about 23 minutes, stirring continuously. Drizzle parsley and remove from heat. Serve the chicken pieces with the topping of capers sauce.

**Nutrition:**
Calories 352
Fat 13.5
Carbohydrates 1.9g
Protein 1.2g

## 303. Slow Cooker Mediterranean Beef Roast

**Preparation Time: 15 Minutes**
**Cooking Time:** 25 Minutes
**Servings: 3**
**Ingredients:**
3 pounds Chuck roast, boneless
2 teaspoons Rosemary
1/2 cup Tomatoes, sundried and chopped
10 cloves Grated garlic
1/2 cup Beef stock
2 tablespoons Balsamic vinegar
1/4 cup Chopped Italian parsley, fresh
1/4 cup Chopped olives
1 teaspoon Lemon zest
1/4 cup Cheese grits
**Directions:**
In the slow cooker, put garlic, sun dried tomatoes, and the beef roast. Add beef stock and Rosemary. Close the cooker and slow cook for 10 hours. After cooking is over, remove the beef, and shred the meet. Discard the fat. Add back the shredded meat to the slow cooker and simmer for 10 minutes. In a small bowl combine lemon zest, parsley, and olives. Cool the mixture until you are ready to serve. Garnish using the refrigerated mix.
Serve it over pasta or egg noodles. Top it with cheese grits.
**Nutrition:**
Calories 314
Fat 19g
Carbohydrate 1g
Protein 32g

## 304. Slow Cooker Mediterranean Beef with Artichokes

**Preparation Time: 15 Minutes**
**Cooking Time:** 25 Minutes
**Servings: 3**
**Ingredients:**
2 pounds Beef for stew
14 ounces Artichoke hearts
1 tablespoon Grape seed oil
1 Diced onion
32 ounces Beef broth
4 cloves Garlic, grated
14 1/2 ounces Tinned tomatoes, diced
15 ounces Tomato sauce
1 teaspoon Dried oregano
1/2 cup Pitted, chopped olives
1 teaspoon Dried parsley
1 teaspoon Dried oregano
1/2 teaspoon Ground cumin
1 teaspoon Dried basil
1 Bay leaf
1/2 teaspoon Salt

**Directions:**
In a large nonstick skillet pour some oil and bring to mediumhigh heat. Roast the beef until it turns brown on both the sides. Transfer the beef into a slow cooker.

Add in beef broth, diced tomatoes, tomato sauce, salt and combine. Pour in beef broth, diced tomatoes, oregano, olives, basil, parsley, bay leaf, and cumin. Combine the mixture thoroughly.

Close and cook on low heat for 7 hours. Discard the bay leaf at the time serving. Serve hot.

**Nutrition:**
Calories 416
Fat 5g
Carbohydrates 14.1g
Protein 29.9g

## 305. Skinny Slow Cooker Mediterranean Style Pot Roast

**Preparation Time: 15 Minutes**
**Cooking Time:** 25 Minutes
**Servings: 3**
**Ingredients:**
4 pounds Eye of round roast
4 cloves Garlic
2 teaspoons Olive oil
1 teaspoon Freshly ground black pepper
1 cup Chopped onions
4 Carrots, chopped
2 teaspoons Dried Rosemary
2 Chopped celery stalks
28 ounces Crushed tomatoes in the can
1 cup Low sodium beef broth
1 cup Red wine
2 teaspoons Salt

**Directions:**
Season the beef roast with salt, garlic, and pepper and set aside. Pour oil in a nonstick skillet and bring to mediumhigh heat. Put the beef into it and roast until it becomes brown on all sides. Now, transfer the roasted beef into a 6quart slow cooker. Add carrots, onion, rosemary, and celery into the skillet. Continue cooking until the onion and vegetable become soft.

Stir in the tomatoes and wine into this vegetable mixture. Add beef broth and tomato mixture into the slow cooker along with the vegetable mixture. Close and cook on low for 8 hours.

Once the meat gets cooked, remove it from the slow cooker and place it on a cutting board and wrap with an aluminum foil. To thicken the sauce, then transfer it into a saucepan and boil it under low heat until it reaches to the required consistency. Discard fats before serving.

**Nutrition:**
Calories 260
Fat 6g
Carbohydrates 8.7g
Protein 37.6g

## 306. Slow Cooker Mediterranean Beef Hoagies

**Preparation Time: 15 Minutes**
**Cooking Time:** 25 Minutes
**Servings: 3**
**Ingredients:**
3 pounds Beef top round roast fatless
1/2 teaspoon Onion powder
1/2 teaspoon Black pepper
3 cups Low sodium beef broth
4 teaspoons Salad dressing mix
1 Bay leaf
1 tablespoon Garlic, minced
2 Red bell peppers, thin strips cut
16 ounces Pepperoncino
8 slices provolone cheese, thin
2 ounces Glutenfree bread
1/2 teaspoon salt

**For seasoning:**
11/2 tablespoon Onion powder
11/2 tablespoon Garlic powder
2 tablespoon Dried parsley
1 tablespoon stevia
1/2 teaspoon Dried thyme
1 tablespoon Dried oregano
2 tablespoons Black pepper
1 tablespoon Salt
6 Cheese slices

**Directions:**
Dry the roast with a paper towel. Combine black pepper, onion powder and salt in a small bowl and rub the mixture over the roast. Place the seasoned roast into a slow cooker.
Add broth, salad dressing mix, bay leaf, and garlic to the slow cooker. Combine it gently. Close and set to low cooking

for 12 hours. After cooking, remove the bay leaf.
Take out the cooked beef and shred the beef meet. Put back the shredded beef and add bell peppers and. Add bell peppers and pepperoncino into the slow cooker. Cover the cooker and low cook for 1 hour. Before serving, top each of the bread with 3 ounces of the meat mixture. Top it with a cheese slice. The liquid gravy can be used as a dip.

**Nutrition:**
Calories 442
Fat 11.5g
Carbohydrates 37g
Protein 49g

## 307. Chicken in TomatoBalsamic Pan Sauce

**Preparation Time: 15 Minutes**
**Cooking Time:** 25 Minutes
**Servings: 3**
**Ingredients:**
2 (8 oz. or 226.7 g each) boneless chicken breasts, skinless
1/2 tsp. salt
1/2 tsp. ground pepper
3 tbsps. extravirgin olive oil
1/2 c. halved cherry tomatoes
2 tbsps. sliced shallot
1/4 c. balsamic vinegar
1 tbsp. minced garlic
1 tbsp. toasted fennel seeds, crushed
1 tbsp. butter

**Directions:**
Slice the chicken breasts into 4 pieces and beat them with a mallet till it reaches a thickness of a 1/4 inch. Use 1/4 teaspoons of pepper and salt to coat the chicken. Heat two tablespoons of oil in a skillet and keep the heat to a medium. Cook the chicken breasts on each side for three

minutes. Place it to a serving plate and cover it with foil to keep it warm.

Add one tablespoon oil, shallot, and tomatoes in a pan and cook till it softens. Add vinegar and boil the mix till the vinegar gets reduced by half. Put fennel seeds, garlic, salt, and pepper and cook for about four minutes. Pull it out from the heat and stir it with butter. Pour this sauce over chicken and serve.

**Nutrition:**
Calories 294
Fat 17g
Carbohydrates 10g
Protein 2g

## 308. Brown Rice, Feta, Fresh Pea, and Mint Salad

**Preparation Time: 15 Minutes**
**Cooking Time:** 25 Minutes
**Servings: 3**
**Ingredients:**
2 c. brown rice
3 c. water
Salt
5 oz. or 141.7 g crumbled feta cheese
2 c. cooked peas
1/2 c. chopped mint, fresh
2 tbsps. olive oil
Salt and pepper
**Directions:**
Place the brown rice, water, and salt into a saucepan over medium heat, cover, and bring to boiling point. Turn the lower heat and allow it to cook until the water has dissolved and the rice is soft but chewy. Leave to cool completely

Add the feta, peas, mint, olive oil, salt, and pepper to a salad bowl with the cooled rice and toss to combine  Serve and enjoy!
**Nutrition:**
Calories 613

Fat 18.2g
Carbohydrates 45g
Protein 12g

## 309. Whole Grain Pita Bread Stuffed with Olives and Chickpeas

**Preparation Time: 15 Minutes**
**Cooking Time:** 25 Minutes
**Servings: 3**
**Ingredients:**
2 wholegrain pita pockets
2 tbsps. olive oil
2 garlic cloves, chopped
1 onion, chopped
1/2 tsp. cumin
10 black olives, chopped
2 c. cooked chickpeas
Salt and pepper
**Directions:**
Slice open the pita pockets and set aside Adjust your heat to medium and set a pan in place. Add in the olive oil and heat.  Mix in the garlic, onion, and cumin to the hot pan and stir as the onions soften and the cumin is fragrant  Add the olives, chickpeas, salt, and pepper and toss everything together until the chickpeas become golden

Set the pan from heat and use your wooden spoon to roughly mash the chickpeas so that some are intact and some are crushed  Heat your pita pockets in the microwave, in the oven, or on a clean pan on the stove

Fill them with your chickpea mixture and enjoy!
**Nutrition:**
Calories 503
Fat 19g
Carbohydrates 14g
Protein 15.7g

## 310. Shish Kebabs

**Preparation Time: 15 Minutes**
**Cooking Time:** 25 Minutes
**Servings: 3**
**Ingredients:**
1/2 cup sugar
1/2 cup reducedsodium soy sauce
1/2 cup ketchup
1 tsp garlic powder
1 tsp ground ginger
1 pounds sirloin steak, cut into 11/2inch cubes
12 small zucchini, cut into 1inch slices
1/4 pound medium fresh mushrooms
1 sweet red/green pepper, cut into 1inch pieces
45 cherry tomatoes, halved
1 small onion, cut into 1inch pieces
1 cup cubed fresh pineapple
**Directions:**
Mix first five ingredients for the marinade.
Place half of the marinade and beef in a large plastic bag; turn to coat and seal the bag, allowing to marinate overnight.

Reserve and cover the remaining marinade.
Thread beef, vegetables, and pineapple on metal or wooden skewers.
Steam, covered, over medium heat until beef reaches desired doneness and vegetables are tender, occasionally turning, 1215 minutes.
Boil the reserved marinade in a small saucepan, stirring occasionally, about 1 minute. Serve with kebabs.
**Nutrition:**
Carbs – 38 G  Fat – 5 G
Protein – 27 G  Calories – 306

## 311. Steamed Steak With Barley Salad
**Preparation Time: 15 Minutes**
**Cooking Time:** 25 Minutes
**Servings: 3**

**Ingredients:**
1 tsp Italian seasoning blend
1/2 pound flank steak, trimmed
1/8 tsp black pepper
1/4 tsp salt
1 cup cooked barley
1/2 (15 oz) can no salt added chickpeas, drained and rinsed
1/4 cup chopped roasted tomatoes
1 cucumber, seeded and diced
1/8 cup chopped fresh basil
1/4 cup lemon juice
1/8 cup crumbled feta
1/8 cup pitted Kalamata olives, chopped
**Directions:**
Heat a Steam pan over mediumhigh or heat a Steam to mediumhigh.
Dry steak with a paper towel and sprinkle both sides with Italian seasoning, pepper and 1/4 tsp salt.
Steam steak 46 minutes for each side or until it reaches desired degree of doneness.
Transfer to a foiled cutting board and allow to rest 5 minutes, then cut into thin strips across the grain.
In a medium bowl, combine remaining ingredients.
**Nutrition:**
Carbs – 48 g  Fat – 23 g
Protein – 28 g
Calories – 508

## 312. Chicken Marsala
**Preparation Time: 15 Minutes**
**Cooking Time:** 25 Minutes
**Servings: 3**
**Ingredients:**
1 pounds boneless skinless chicken breasts, pounded 1/4" thick
1/2 Tbsp allpurpose flour
salt and black pepper, to taste
1 Tbsp olive oil
1/2 Tbsp unsalted butter, divided

4 oz button mushrooms, sliced

11/2 Tbsp shallots, finely chopped

2 cloves garlic, minced

1/2 cup chicken broth

1/2 cup dry Marsala wine

1/2 cup heavy cream

1 tsp chopped fresh thyme

1 Tbsp chopped fresh parsley, for serving

**Directions:**

Add flour, 3/4 tsp salt, and 1/4 tsp pepper in a Ziplock bag.

Place chicken in the bag and seal it. Shake to coat evenly. Set aside.

Over mediumhigh, heat oil and 2 Tbsps butter in a large skillet.

Place chicken in the pan, shaking off excess flour, and cook for 34 minutes per side until golden and barely cooked through. Transfer to a plate and set aside.

Melt 1 Tbsp butter in the pan.

Add mushrooms and cook for 34 minutes, occasionally stirring until they begin to brown.

Add shallots, garlic, and 1/4 tsp of salt. Cook for 12 minutes more.

Add broth, heavy cream, Marsala, thyme, 1/4 tsp salt, and 1/8 tsp pepper.

Let it boil, turn to medium, and cook for 1015 minutes until it is reduced by half and slightly thickened.

Back chicken back to the pan, along with any juices that accumulated on the plate. Reduce to low and simmer for 23 minutes more. Sprinkle with parsley, if using.

**Nutrition:**

Carbs – 15 g

Fat – 8 g

Protein – 4 g

Calories – 140

## 313. Greek Chicken Pitas with Cucumber & OrzoFeta Salad

**Preparation Time: 15 Minutes**

**Cooking Time:** 25 Minutes

**Servings: 3**

**Ingredients:**

2 boneless, skinless chicken breasts

3 oz orzo pasta

2 pitas

1/2 cup plain Greek yogurt

2 cloves garlic, smashed

1 cucumber, peeled and diced

1 lemon, quartered

1 bunch mint leaves

1 bunch oregano, stems removed

1/4 cup crumbled feta cheese

1 oz kalamata olives, smashed

**Directions:**

Heat a pot filled with salted water to boiling on high.

Pat dry chicken with paper towels and season with salt and pepper.

In a pan, heat oil on medium high.

Add chicken and cook for 4 6 minutes per side, until cooked through. Remove to a cutting board.

To make dressing, mix oregano, half garlic paste, 2 lemon wedges juice, and drizzle with olive oil in a bowl. Season with salt and pepper.

When cool enough, slice cooked chicken. Add to the dressing bowl and toss to coat.

Mix yogurt, half cucumber, half mint, lemon juice, and garlic paste in a bowl. Add oil, salt and pepper. Stir to combine.

Heat the pan on medium high.

Warm pitas – one at one time – for 1 minute per side. Transfer to a cutting board and cut in half.

Add, olives, remaining cucumber, cheese, remaining mint to the pot of cooked pasta, and drizzle with oil. Stir to combine.

Transfer to a serving plate and fill halved pitas with cucumber chicken.

**Nutrition:**

Carbs – 83 g

Fat – 23 g

Protein – 51 g

Calories – 750

## 314. Greek Chicken Gyros

**Preparation Time: 15 Minutes**

**Cooking Time:** 25 Minutes

**Servings: 3**

**Ingredients:**

1/2 pounds boneless chicken thighs

1/2 red onion

2 pitas

1/2 cup Tatziki sauce

FOR GYRO MARINADE

3/4 Tbsp finely chopped garlic.

3/4 Tbsp lemon juice

1/2 tsp whole pepper corns

1/3 cup extravirgin olive oil

3/4 Tbsp paprika powder

1 Tbsp dried rosemary

1 Tbsp whole coriander seeds

1 Tbsp dried red chili flakes

coarse sea salt to taste

**Directions:**

Preheat oven at 375°F.

Pound each chicken thigh until 1/2" thick with a meat mallet. Set aside.

Add paprika, coriander, peppercorns, rosemary, chili flakes, and salt in a mortar and pestle to a semicoarse powder.

Add chopped garlic and grind it until garlic blends with the rest of spice blend.

Pour in oil and lemon juice and mix well.

Add marinade to chicken thighs and mix until all the chicken thighs are evenly coated.

Wrap container, using a cling film, and leave overnight in the fridge to marinate.

Take a large onion stump and stick a bamboo skewer in the center of stump to create a vertical pole.

Put each chicken thigh and skewer them individually in the homemade vertical rotisserie.

Bake for 1 hour by placing vertical rotisserie over a cookie tray.

Let it cool for 15 minutes. Shave chicken meat and serve with Tzatziki sauce.

**Nutrition:**

Carbs – 15 g

Fat – 8 g

Protein – 4 g

Calories – 140

## 315. Greek Chicken in TomatoKotopoulo Kokkinisto

**Preparation Time: 15 Minutes**

**Cooking Time:** 25 Minutes

**Servings: 3**

**Ingredients:**

1/2 pound chicken in pieces

1/2 onion, diced

1 Tbsp olive oil

1 minced garlic clove

1/4 cup water

5 ounces diced tomatoes

1 cinnamon stick

12 allspice berries

1 bay leaf

salt and pepper, to taste

**Directions:**

Heat olive oil and cook chicken pieces on both sides for 45 minutes in a large deep pan.

Set chicken aside and add onion. Cook until soft. Add garlic and cook for 1 minute.

Add 1/3 cup water, tomato, cinnamon stick, bay leaf, allspice, salt, and pepper and mix well. Add chicken and blend. Cover and simmer until cooked, for 45 minutes.

Serve warm with preferable sidedish.

**Nutrition:**
Carbs – 3 g
Fat – 16 g
Protein – 19 g
Calories – 226

## 316. Greek Chicken and Potatoes
**Preparation Time: 15 Minutes**
**Cooking Time:** 25 Minutes
**Servings: 3**
**Ingredients:**
1 whole chicken
2 lemons juice
1/3 cup extravirgin olive oil
2 Tbsp dried oregano
11 cloves garlic, minced
4 medium potatoes, quartered
salt and pepper, to taste
**Directions:**
Preheat oven to 350°F. Cover a sheet pan with parchment paper.

Place chicken on a cutting board breastsidedown. Using a knife, cut chicken in half along the backbone. Turn it over and cut through the center of breastbone. Divide two halves and lay them on prepared pan skinsideup.

Squeeze 1 lemon juice onto chicken and rub it into whole chicken. Coat with olive oil and rub again to coat the skin. Season chicken with salt and pepper. Sprinkle 1 Tbsp oregano and half garlic over chicken.

Put potatoes in a large bowl. Add the rest olive oil, garlic, oregano, and 1 lemon juice, salt, and pepper. Toss to coat.

Arrange potatoes on the sheet pan around the chicken.

Roast for 1 hour 15 minutes until chicken is cooked through, and both are golden and crispy.

**Nutrition:**
Carbs – 41 g
Fat – 12 g
Protein – 44 g
Calories – 468

## 317. Mediterranean Sauteed Chicken
**Preparation Time: 15 Minutes**
**Cooking Time:** 25 Minutes
**Servings: 3**
**Ingredients:**
1 tsp olive oil
1 Tbsp white wine
2 skinless, boneless chicken breast halves
2 cloves garlic, minced
1/4 cup diced onion
2 cups cherry tomatoes
1/4 cup white wine
1 tsp chopped fresh thyme
3 tsp fresh basil
1/4 cup kalamata olives
1/8 cup chopped fresh parsley
Salt and pepper, to taste
**Directions:**
Heat 2 Tbsps white wine and the oil in a large skillet over mediumlow heat.

Add chicken and saute about 46 minutes each side, until goldenbrown. Remove chicken from the skillet. Set aside.

Saute garlic in pan for 30 seconds, then add onion and saute for 3 minutes.

Add cherry tomatoes and bring to a boil.

Lower the heat and add the rest white wine. Simmer approximately 10 minutes.

Add basil and thyme and simmer for 5 minutes.

Put the chicken back in the skillet and cover.

Cook over the low heat until the chicken is cooked and no longer pink inside.

Add parsley and olives to the skillet and cook for 1 minute.

Season with pepper and salt to taste.

**Nutrition:**

Carbs – 7 g

Fat – 6 g

Protein – 29 g

Calories – 222

## 318. Chicken Stuffed with Cheese

**Preparation Time: 15 Minutes**

**Cooking Time:** 25 Minutes

**Servings: 3**

**Ingredients:**

2 chicken boneless, skinless breasts, pounded thin

1/4 cup feta cheese

2 ounces cream cheese, softened

1/2 tsp garlic powder

1 Tbsp melted butter

1 tsp dried dill weed

Salt and pepper, to taste

**Directions:**

Preheat oven to 350°F.

Beat the cream cheese in a large bowl until smooth.

Add the feta cheese, garlic powder, and dill weed. Beat until creamy, smooth texture.

On each breast put 1/2 of the filling, then roll and tie the breasts with the cooking string to seal.

Brush every breast with melted butter and sprinkle with pepper and salt.

Bake uncovered for 20 minutes or until the juices run clear.

**Nutrition:**

Carbs – 3 g

Fat – 22 g

Protein – 33 g

Calories – 339

## 319. Greek Lemony Chicken Skewers

**Preparation Time: 15 Minutes**

**Cooking Time:** 25 Minutes

**Servings: 3**

**Ingredients:**

1 pound boneless, skinless chicken breasts

1 Tbsp dried oregano leaves

2 large cloves garlic, minced

1/2 tsp grated lemon rind

3 Tbsps lemon juice

Pinch freshly ground pepper

For Tzatziki sauce:

2/3 cup 0% Greek yogurt

1/3 cup shredded cucumber, squeezed dry

1 small clove garlic, minced

1 Tbsp fresh dill, chopped

1/2 tsp lemon zest

**Directions:**

Cut chicken breasts into 1inch strips and chop every strip into 11/2inch chunks.

Place in a bowl and add garlic, oregano, pepper, lemon rind, and juice. Stir to coat well. Cover and refrigerate about 30 minutes.

In a separate bowl, stir yogurt, cucumber, dill, garlic, and lemon zest until combined. Cover and refrigerate 24 hours.

Preheat broiler to high, or if using the Steam, preheat to mediumhigh.

Skewer chicken onto 4 metal or soaked wooden skewers.

If using a broiler, place skewers on a foillined baking sheet and place sheet in the oven, about 6 inches from broiler. Turn once after 8 minutes or until goldenbrowned and no longer pink inside.

If using a Steam, place chicken skewers on greased Steam over medium heat for about 10 minutes. Turn once.

Garnish with tzatziki sauce.

**Nutrition:**

Carbs – 2 g

Fat – 2 g

Protein – 32 g

Calories – 166

## 320. Creole Spaghetti

**Preparation Time: 15 Minutes**

**Cooking Time:** 25 Minutes

**Servings: 3**

**Ingredients:**

1 extra virgin olive oil

11/4 lbs. ground beef (85% lean)

1/4 lb country ham, cut into 1/4" pieces (about 3/4 cup)

1 can tomato sauce

1/2 cup sofrito

1/2 Tbsp minced garlic

1/2 Tbsp sugar

1/4 tsp ground cumin

1/4 tsp oregano

1/4 packet sazon with coriander & annatto

1/4 cup manzanillo olives stuffed with minced pimientos, chopped

1/2 cup finely chopped fresh cilantro, divided

1/2 tsp. adobo allpurpose seasoning with pepper

1/2 lb. spaghetti

parmesan cheese, to taste

**Directions:**
Over mediumhigh, heat olive oil in a skillet and add beef. Cook until browned, about 6 minutes.

Transfer the beef over to the plate.

Reheat the pan over medium heat and add the ham. Cook, stirring occasionally, for about 4 minutes, until the ham is golden brown.

Add tomato sauce, garlic, sugar, cumin, oregano and sazon to the pan. Cook until the mixture of tomato sauce starts to bubble.

Stir in reserved beef, olives, 1/8 cup coriander and Adobo. Simmer, stirring occasionally, until sauce thickens and flavours, about 8 minutes longer. Stir in the remaining coriander.

Cook spaghetti according to the manufacture's instructions.

Strain pasta, reserve 11/2 cups water.

Add reserved pasta water and spaghetti to skillet with sauce over mediumhigh heat.

Toss spaghetti with sauce for 3 minutes, using tongs.

Serve with Parmesan cheese.

**Nutrition:**
Carbs – 57 g
Fat – 8 g
Protein – 4 g
Calories – 413

## 321. Honey Almond Chicken Tenders

**Preparation Time: 15 Minutes**
**Cooking Time:** 25 Minutes
**Servings: 3**
**Ingredients:**
1 Tablespoon Honey, Raw
1 Tablespoon Dijon Mustard
1 Cup Almonds
Sea Salt & Black Pepper to Taste
1 lb. Chicken Breast Tenders, Boneless & Skinless

**Directions:**
Start by heating your oven to 425, and then get out a baking sheet. Line it with parchment paper, and then put a cooking rack on it. Spray your cooling rack down with nonstick cooking spray.

Get out a bowl and combine your mustard and honey. Season with salt and pepper, and then add in your chicken. Make sure it's well coated and place it to the side.

Use a knife and chop your almonds. You can also use a food processor. You want them to roughly be the same size as sunflower seeds. Press your chicken into the almonds, and then lay it on your cooking rack.

Bake for fifteen to twenty minutes. Your chicken should be cooked all the way through.

**Nutrition:**
Calories: 263
Protein: 31 Grams
Fat: 12 Grams
Carbs: 9 Grams

## 322. Parsley Chicken with Potatoes

**Preparation Time: 15 Minutes**
**Cooking Time:** 25 Minutes
**Servings: 3**
**Ingredients:**
1 1/2 lb. Chicken Thighs, Boneless, Skinless & Cut into 1 Inch Cubes
1 Tablespoons Olive Oil
1 1/2 lbs. Gold Potatoes, Unpeeled & Cubed
2 Cloves Garlic, Minced
1/4 Cup Dry White Wine
1 Cup Chicken Broth, Low Sodium
Sea Salt & Black Pepper to Taste
1 Tablespoon Dijon Mustard
1 Cup Italian Parsley, Fresh & Chopped

1 Tablespoon Lemon Juice, Fresh

**Directions:**
Start by patting your chicken dry using paper towels, and then get out a large skillet. Place it over mediumhigh heat and heat up your oil. Add in your chicken, and cook for five minutes. Stir once the chicken is browned on one side. Remove it from pan, and place it on the plate. Leave the skillet overheat. Add in the potatoes, cooking for five minutes. Stir once they're crispy and golden on one side, and then push them to the side. Add in your garlic and cook while stirring for one minute. Add in your wine and cook for a minute more. It should be nearly evaporated. Add in the mustard, chicken broth, and chicken back into the skillet. Season with salt and pepper. Turn the heat up to high, and then bring it all to a boil.

Cover the skillet and reduce the heat to mediumlow. Cook for an additional ten to twelve minutes.

During the lastminute stir in your parsley, and then remove it from heat. Stir in your lemon juice before serving.

**Nutrition:**
Calories: 241
Protein: 29 Grams
Fat: 4 Grams
Carbs: 20 Grams

## 323. Baked Balsamic Fish
**Preparation Time: 15 Minutes**
**Cooking Time:** 25 Minutes
**Servings: 3**
**Ingredients:**
1 tablespoon balsamic vinegar
2 1/2 cups green beans
1pint cherry or grape tomatoes
4 (4ounce each) fish fillets, such as cod or tilapia
2 tablespoons olive oil

**Directions:**
Preheat an oven to 400 degrees. Grease two baking sheets with some olive oil or olive oil spray. Arrange 2 fish fillets on each sheet. In a mixing bowl, pour olive oil and vinegar. Combine to mix well with each other. Mix green beans and tomatoes. Combine to mix well with each other. Combine both mixtures well with each other. Add mixture equally over fish fillets. Bake for 68 minutes, until fish opaque and easy to flake. Serve warm.

**Nutrition:**
Calories 229
Fat 13g
Carbohydrates 8g
Protein 2.5g

## 324. MediterraneanSpiced Swordfish
**Preparation Time: 15 Minutes**
**Cooking Time:** 25 Minutes
**Servings: 3**
**Ingredients:**
4 (7 ounces each) swordfish steaks
1/2 teaspoon ground black pepper
12 cloves of garlic, peeled
3/4 teaspoon salt
1 1/2 teaspoon ground cumin
1 teaspoon paprika
1 teaspoon coriander
3 tablespoons lemon juice
1/3 cup olive oil

**Directions:**
Using food processor, incorporate all the ingredients except for swordfish. Seal the lid and blend to make a smooth mixture. Pat dry fish steaks; coat equally with the prepared spice mixture.

Situate them over an aluminum foil, cover and refrigerator for 1 hour. Prep a griddle pan over high heat, cook oil.

Put fish steaks; stircook for 56 minutes per side until cooked through and evenly browned.  Serve warm.

**Nutrition:**
Calories 275
Fat 17g
Carbohydrates 5g
Protein 0.5g

### 325. Sweet and Sour Salmon
**Preparation Time: 15 Minutes**
**Cooking Time:** 25 Minutes
**Servings: 3**
**Ingredients:**
4 (8ounce) salmon filets
1/2 cup balsamic vinegar
1 tablespoon honey
Black pepper and salt, to taste
1 tablespoon olive oil
**Directions:**
Combine honey and vinegar. Combine to mix well with each other.
Season fish fillets with the black pepper (ground) and sea salt; brush with honey glaze. Take a medium saucepan or skillet, add oil. Heat over medium heat.  Add salmon fillets and stircook until medium rare in center and lightly browned for 34 minutes per side.  Serve warm.

**Nutrition:**
Calories 481 Fat 16g
Carbohydrates 24g
Protein1.5g

### 326. CitrusBaked Fish
**Preparation Time: 15 Minutes**
**Cooking Time:** 25 Minutes
**Servings: 3**
**Ingredients:**
1/4 teaspoon kosher or sea salt
1 tablespoon extravirgin olive oil
1 tablespoon orange juice
4 (4ounce) tilapia fillets, with or without skin

1/4 cup chopped red onion
1 avocado, pitted, skinned, and sliced
**Directions:**
Take a baking dish of 9inch; add olive oil, orange juice, and salt. Combine well.  Add fish fillets and coat well. Add onions over fish fillets.
Cover with a plastic wrap.  Microwave for 3 minutes until fish is cooked well and easy to flake. Serve warm with sliced avocado on top.

**Nutrition:**
Calories 231
Fat 9g
Carbohydrates 8g
Protein 2.5g

### 327. LemonGarlic Shrimp Zoodles
**Preparation Time: 15 Minutes**
**Cooking Time:** 25 Minutes
**Servings: 3**
**Ingredients:**
2 tablespoons chopped parsley
2 teaspoons minced garlic
1 teaspoon salt
1/2 teaspoon black pepper
2 medium zucchinis, spiralized
3/4 pounds medium shrimp, peeled & deveined
1 tablespoon olive oil
1 lemon, juiced and zested
**Directions:**
Take a medium saucepan or skillet, add oil, lemon juice, lemon zest. Heat over medium heat.  Add shrimps and stircook 1 minute per side.
Sauté garlic and red pepper flakes for 1 more minute.  Add Zoodles and stir gently; cook for 3 minutes until cooked to satisfaction.  Season well, serve warm with parsley on top.
**Nutrition:**
Calories 329 Fat 12g
Carbohydrates 11g

Protein 3g

## 328. OnePan Asparagus Trout

**Preparation Time: 15 Minutes**
**Cooking Time:** 25 Minutes
**Servings: 3**
**Ingredients:**
2 pounds trout fillets
1pound asparagus
Salt and ground white pepper, to taste
1 tablespoon olive oil
1 garlic clove, finely minced
1 scallion, thinly sliced (green and white part)
4 medium golden potatoes, thinly sliced
2 Roma tomatoes, chopped
8 pitted Kalamata olives, chopped
1 large carrot, thinly sliced
2 tablespoons dried parsley
1/4 cup ground cumin
2 tablespoons paprika
1 tablespoon vegetable bouillon seasoning
1/2 cup dry white wine
**Directions:**
In a mixing bowl, add fish fillets, white pepper and salt. Combine to mix well with each other. Take a medium saucepan or skillet, add oil. Heat over medium heat. Add asparagus, potatoes, garlic, white part scallion, and stircook until become softened for 45 minutes. Add tomatoes, carrot and olives; stircook for 67 minutes until turn tender. Add cumin, paprika, parsley, bouillon seasoning, and salt. Stir mixture well.
Mix in white wine and fish fillets. Over low heat, cover and simmer mixture for about 6 minutes until fish is easy to flake, stir in between. Serve warm with green scallions on top.

**Nutrition:**
Calories 303
Fat 17g
Carbohydrates 37g
Protein 6g

## 329. *Olive Tuna*

**Preparation Time: 15 Minutes**
**Cooking Time:** 25 Minutes
**Servings: 3**
**Ingredients:**
1 cup chopped onion
3 garlic cloves, minced
1 (2.25ounce) can sliced olives, drained
1pound kale, chopped
3 tablespoons extravirgin olive oil
1/4 cup capers
1/4 teaspoon crushed red pepper
2 teaspoons sugar
1 (15ounce) can cannellini beans
2 (6ounce) cans tuna in olive oil, undrained
1/4 teaspoon black pepper
1/4 teaspoon kosher or sea salt
**Directions:**
Soak kale in boiling water for 2 minutes; drain and set aside. Take a mediumlarge cooking pot or stock pot, heat oil over medium heat. Add onion and stircook until become translucent and softened. Add garlic and stircook until become fragrant for 1 minute.
Add olives, capers, and red pepper, and stircook for 1 minute. Mix in cooked kale and sugar. Over low heat, cover and simmer mixture for about 810 minutes, stir in between. Add tuna, beans, pepper, and salt. Stir well and serve warm.
**Nutrition:**
Calories 242
Fat| 11g
Carbohydrates 24g

Protein 7g

## 330. RosemaryCitrus Shrimps

**Preparation Time: 15 Minutes**
**Cooking Time:** 25 Minutes
**Servings: 3**
**Ingredients:**

1 large orange, zested and peeled
3 garlic cloves, minced
1 1/2 pounds raw shrimp, shells and tails removed
3 tablespoons olive oil
1 tablespoon chopped thyme
1 tablespoon chopped rosemary
1/4 teaspoon black pepper
1/4 teaspoon kosher or sea salt

**Directions:**

Take a ziptop plastic bag, add orange zest, shrimps, 2 tablespoons olive oil, garlic, thyme, rosemary, salt, and black pepper. Shake well and set aside to marinate for 5 minutes.

Take a medium saucepan or skillet, add 1 tablespoon olive oil. Heat over medium heat. Add shrimps and stircook for 23 minutes per side until totally pink and opaque. Slice orange into bitesized wedges and add in a serving plate. Add shrimps and combine well. Serve fresh.

**Nutrition:**

Calories 187
Fat 7g
Carbohydrates 6g
Protein 0.5g

## 331. PanSeared Asparagus Salmon

**Preparation Time: 15 Minutes**
**Cooking Time:** 25 Minutes
**Servings: 3**
**Ingredients:**

8.8ounce bunch asparagus
2 small salmon fillets
1 1/2 teaspoon salt
1 teaspoon black pepper
1 tablespoon olive oil
1 cup hollandaise sauce, lowcarb

**Directions:**

Season well the salmon fillets. Take a medium saucepan or skillet, add oil. Heat over medium heat.

Add salmon fillets and stircook until evenly seared and cooked well for 45 minutes per side. Add asparagus and stir cook for 45 more minutes. Serve warm with hollandaise sauce on top.

**Nutrition:**

Calories 565
Fat 7g
Carbohydrates 8g
Protein 2.5g

## 332. Creamy Leek Shrimp Stew

**Preparation Time: 15 Minutes**
**Cooking Time:** 25 Minutes
**Servings: 3**
**Ingredients:**

1pound medium shrimp, peeled and deveined
1 leek, both whites and light green parts, sliced
1 medium fennel bulb, chopped
2 tablespoons olive oil
3 stalks celery, chopped
1 clove garlic, minced
Sea salt and ground pepper to taste
4 cups vegetable or chicken broth
1 tablespoon fennel seeds
2 tablespoons light cream
Juice of 1 lemon

**Directions:**

Take a mediumlarge cooking pot or Dutch oven, heat oil over medium heat. Add celery, leek, and fennel and stircook for about 15 minutes, until vegetables are softened and browned. Add garlic; season with black pepper and sea salt to taste. Add fennel seed and stir.

Pour broth and bring to a boil. Over low heat, simmer mixture for about 20 minutes, stir in between. Add shrimp and cook until just pink for 3 minutes. Mix in cream and lemon juice; serve warm.

**Nutrition:**
Calories 174
Fat 5g
Carbohydrates 9.5g
Protein 2g

### 333. Salmon and Vegetable Quinoa
**Preparation Time: 15 Minutes**
**Cooking Time:** 25 Minutes
**Servings: 3**
**Ingredients:**
1 cup uncooked quinoa
1 teaspoon of salt, divided in half
3/4 cup cucumbers, seeds removed, diced
1 cup of cherry tomatoes, halved
1/4 cup red onion, minced
4 fresh basil leaves, cut in thin slices
Zest from one lemon
1/4 teaspoon black pepper
1 teaspoon cumin
1/2 teaspoon paprika
4 (5oz.) salmon fillets
8 lemon wedges
1/4 cup fresh parsley, chopped
**Directions:**
To a mediumsized saucepan, add the quinoa, 2 cups of water, and 1/2 teaspoons of the salt. Heat these until the water is boiling, then lower the temperature until it is simmering. Cover the pan and let it cook 20 minutes or as long as the quinoa package instructs. Turn off the burner under the quinoa and allow it to sit,

covered, for at least another 5 minutes before serving.

Right before serving, mix onion, tomatoes, cucumbers, basil leaves, and lemon zest to the quinoa. In the meantime (while the quinoa cooks), prepare the salmon. Turn on the oven broiler to high and make sure a rack is in the lower part of the oven. To a small bowl, add the following components: black pepper, 1/2 teaspoon of the salt, cumin, and paprika. Stir them together.

Place foil over the top of a glass or aluminum baking sheet, then spray it with nonstick cooking spray. Place salmon fillets on the foil. Scour the spice mixture over the surface of each fillet (about 1/2 teaspoons of the spice mixture per fillet). Add the lemon wedges to the pan edges near the salmon.

Cook the salmon under the broiler for 810 minutes. Your goal is for the salmon to flake apart easily with a fork. Sprinkle the salmon with the parsley, then serve it with the lemon wedges and vegetable parsley. Enjoy!

**Nutrition:**
385 Calories
12.5g Fat
32.5g Carbohydrates
35.5g Protein

### 334. Gnocchi with Shrimp
**Preparation Time: 15 Minutes**
**Cooking Time:** 25 Minutes
**Servings: 3**
**Ingredients:**
1/2 lb. Shrimp, Peeled & Deveined
1/4 Cup Shallots, Sliced
1/2 Tablespoon + 1 Teaspoon Olive Oil
8 Ounces Shelf Stable Gnocchi
1/2 Bunch Asparagus, Cut into Thirds

3 Tablespoons Parmesan Cheese
1 Tablespoon Lemon Juice, Fresh
1/3 Cup Chicken Broth
Sea Salt & Black Pepper to Taste
**Directions:**
Start by heating a half a tablespoon of oil over medium heat, and then add in your gnocchi. Cook while stirring often until they turn plump and golden. This will take from seven to ten minutes. Place them in a bowl.

Heat your remaining teaspoon of oil with your shallots, cooking until they begin to brown. Make sure to stir, but this will take two minutes. Stir in the broth before adding your asparagus. Cover, and cook for three to four minutes.

Stir in shrimp, seasoning with salt and pepper. Cook until they are pink and cooked through, which will take roughly four minutes.

Return the gnocchi to the skillet with lemon juice, cooking for another two minutes. Stir well, and then remove it from heat.

Sprinkle with parmesan, and let it stand for two minutes. Your cheese should melt. Serve warm.

**Nutrition:**
342 calories
11g fats
9g carbohydrates
38g protein

## 335. Seafood & Avocado
**Preparation Time: 15 Minutes**
**Cooking Time:** 25 Minutes
**Servings: 3**
**Ingredients:**
2 lbs. Salmon, Cooked & Chopped
2 lbs. Shrimp, Cooked & Chopped
1 Cup Avocado, Chopped
1 Cup Mayonnaise
4 Tablespoons Lime Juice, Fresh

2 Cloves Garlic
1 Cup Sour Cream
Sea Salt & Black Pepper to Taste
1/2 Red Onion, Minced
1 Cup Cucumber, Chopped
**Directions:**
Start by getting out a bowl and combine your garlic, salt, pepper, onion, mayonnaise, sour cream and lime juice,

Get out a different bowl and mix together your salmon, shrimp, cucumber, and avocado.

Add the mayonnaise mixture to your shrimp, and then allow it to sit for twenty minutes in the fridge before serving.

**Nutrition:**
Calories: 394
Protein: 27 Grams
Fat: 30 Grams
Carbs: 3 Grams

## 336. Easy Steamed Fish
**Preparation Time: 15 Minutes**
**Cooking Time:** 25 Minutes
**Servings: 3**
**Ingredients:**
4 Lemons
4 Catfish Fillets, 4 Ounces Each
1 Tablespoon Olive Oil
Sea Salt & Black Pepper to Taste
**Directions:**
Pat your fish dry with paper towels, and low it to stand at room temperature for ten minutes. Coat the Steam with cooking spray, and preheat it to 400 degrees.

Cut one of the lemons in half, and then set half of it aside. Slice one half into 1/4 inch slices. Get out a bowl and squeeze a tablespoon of juice from the reserved half.

Mix your lemon juice and oil in a bowl,

and brush your fish down with it. Season with salt and pepper.

Place the lemon slices on the Steam, and place your fish fillets on each one. Turn the fish halfway through, and serve with lemon.

**Nutrition:**
Calories: 147
Protein: 22 Grams
Fat: 5 Grams
Carbs: 4 Grams

## 337. Cod & Green Bean Dinner

**Preparation Time: 15 Minutes**
**Cooking Time:** 25 Minutes
**Servings: 3**
**Ingredients:**
2 Tablespoons Olive Oil
1 Tablespoon Balsamic Vinegar
4 Cod Fillets, 4 Ounces Each
2 1/2 Cups Green Beans
1 Pint Cherry Grapes
**Directions:**
Start by heating your oven to 400, and get out two rimmed baking sheets. Coat them with nonstick cooking spray.

Get out a bowl and whisk your vinegar and oil together before setting it to the side.
Place two pieces of fish on each baking sheet.
Get out a bowl and combine your tomatoes and beans. Pour the oil and vinegar over it, and toss to coat. Pour half of the green bean mixture over the fish on one baking sheet and the remaining fish and green beans on the other.
Turn the fish over, and coat it with the oil mixture.
Bake for five to eight minutes.
**Nutrition:**
Calories; 193

Protein: 23 Grams
Fat: 8 Grams
Carbs: 8 Grams

## 338. Salmon Skillet

**Preparation Time: 15 Minutes**
**Cooking Time:** 25 Minutes
**Servings: 3**
**Ingredients:**
2 Cloves Garlic, Minced
1 Tablespoons Olive Oil
1 Teaspoon Smoked Paprika
12 Ounce Jar Roasted Red Pepper, Chopped & Drained
1 Pinch Grapes, Quartered
Sea Salt & Black Pepper to Taste
1 Tablespoon Water
1 lb. Salmon Fillet, Skinless & Chopped into 8 Pieces
1 Tablespoon Lemon Juice, Fresh
**Directions:**
Start by getting out a skillet, and place it over medium heat to heat your oil.
Once your oil is hot adding in your garlic and smoked paprika. Stir often and cook for a full minute.
Add in your roasted red peppers, tomatoes, water, salt and pepper. Turn it to mediumhigh heat, and bring it to a simmer. Allow it to cook for three minutes, and occasionally stir and smash the tomatoes.
Add in the salmon, and spoon the sauce over it.
Cook while covered for ten to twelve minutes.
Drizzle with lemon juice before serving.
**Nutrition:**
Calories: 289
Protein: 31 Grams Fat: 13 Grams
Carbs: 10 Grams

## 339. Mediterranean Shrimp Salad

**Preparation Time: 15 Minutes**
**Cooking Time:** 25 Minutes
**Servings: 3**
**Ingredients:**
1 1/2 lbs. Shrimp, Cleaned & Cooked
2 Celery Stalks, Fresh
1 Onion
2 Green Onions
4 Eggs, Boiled
3 Potatoes, Cooked
3 Tablespoons Mayonnaise
Sea Salt & Black Pepper to Taste
**Directions:**
Start by slicing your potatoes and chopping your celery.
Slice your eggs, and season. Mix everything together.
Put your shrimp over the eggs, and then serve with onion and green onions.
**Nutrition:**
Calories: 207
Protein: 17 Grams
Fat: 6 Grams
Carbs: 20 Grams

## 340. Kale & Tuna Bowl

**Preparation Time: 15 Minutes**
**Cooking Time:** 25 Minutes
**Servings: 3**
**Ingredients:**
1 lb. Kale, Chopped
3 Tablespoons Olive Oil
2.25 Ounces Olives, Canned & Drained
3 Cloves Garlic, Minced
1 Cup Onion, Chopped
1/4 Cup Capers
1/4 Teaspoon Crushed Red Pepper
2 Teaspoons Sugar
2 Cans Tuna in Olive Oil, Undrained & 6 Ounces Each1
15 Ounce Can Cannellini Beans, Drained & Rinsed
Sea Salt & Black Pepper to Taste

**Directions:**
Get out a large stockpot and fill it three quarters full of water. Bring it to a boil and cook your kale for two minutes. Drain in a colander before setting it aside.
Place your emp ty pot over medium heat, and then add in your oil. Add in your onion, and cook for four minutes. Stir often and cook your garlic for a minute more. Stir often, and then add the olives, crushed red pepper, capers, and cook for a full minute. Stir often, and add your kale and sugar in. stir well, and cook for eight minutes covered.
Remove from heat, and mix in your tuna, pepper, salt, and beans. Serve warm.
**Nutrition:**
Calories: 265
Protein: 16 Grams
Fat: 12 Grams
Carbs: 26 Grams

## 341. Salmon Salad Wraps

**Preparation Time: 15 Minutes**
**Cooking Time:** 25 Minutes
**Servings: 3**
**Ingredients:**
1 lb. Salmon Fillet, Coked & Flaked
1/2 Cup Carrots, Diced
1/2 Cup Celery, Diced
3 Tablespoons Red Onion, Diced
3 Tablespoons Dill, Fresh & Diced
2 Tablespoons Capers
1 Tablespoons Aged Balsamic Vinegar
1 1/2 Tablespoons Olive Oil
Sea Salt & Black Pepper to Taste
4 Whole Wheat Flatbread Wraps
**Directions:**
Get out a bowl and mix your carrots, dill, celery, salmon, red onions, oil, vinegar, pepper, capers and salt together.

Divide between flatbread, and fold up to serve.

**Nutrition:**
Calories: 336
Protein: 32 Grams
Fat: 16 Grams
Carbs: 23 Grams

## 342. Tuna Sandwiches
**Preparation Time: 15 Minutes**
**Cooking Time:** 25 Minutes
**Servings: 3**
**Ingredients:**
3 Tablespoons Lemon Juice, Fresh
2 Tablespoons Olive Oil
Sea Salt & Black Pepper to Taste
1 Clove Garlic, Minced
5 Ounces Canned Tuna, Drained
Ounce Canned Olives, Sliced
1/2 Cup Fennel, Fresh & Chopped
8 Slices Whole Grain Bread

**Directions:**
Start by getting out a bowl and whisk your lemon juice, garlic, pepper and oil before adding in your fennel, olive sand tuna. Use a fork to separate it into chunks before mixing everything together.
Divide this between four slices of bread, and serve.

**Nutrition:**
Calories: 347
Protein: 25 Grams
Fat: 17 Grams
Carbs: 27 Grams

## 343. Garlic & Orange Shrimp
**Preparation Time: 15 Minutes**
**Cooking Time:** 25 Minutes
**Servings: 3**
**Ingredients:**
3 Cloves Garlic, Minced
Sea Salt & Black Pepper to taste
1 1/2 lbs. Shrimp, Fresh & Raw, Deshelled & Tails Removed

1 Tablespoon Thyme, Fresh & Chopped
1 Tablespoon Rosemary, Fresh & Chopped
3 Tablespoons Olive Oil, Divided
1 Orange, Large

**Directions:**
Zest your orange, and then get out a zipper top bag. Combine your zest with two tablespoons of oil and rosemary. Add in your garlic, pepper, salt and thyme. Add in your shrimp, and seal. Massage the shrimp into the seasoning before setting it to the side.
Heat a Steam, and then brush the remaining oil onto your shrimp.
Cook for four to six minutes in a Steam pan, and flip halfway through. Transfer to a serving bowl, and then chop your orange and serve with your shrimp.

**Nutrition:**
Calories: 190
Protein: 24 Grams
Fat: 8 Grams
Carbs: 4 Grams

## 344. Scallops with Peppers
**Preparation Time: 15 Minutes**
**Cooking Time:** 25 Minutes
**Servings: 3**
**Ingredients:**
1/3 Cup Olive Oil
1 Can (2 Ounces) Anchovy Fillets, Minced
1 lb. Sea Scallops, Large
1 Red Bell Pepper, Large & Chopped
1 Red Onion, Sliced Thin
1 Teaspoons Lime Zest
1 Orange Bell Pepper, Chopped
1 1/2 Teaspoons Lemon Zest
Sea Salt & Black Pepper to Taste
8 Sprigs Parsley, Fresh

**Directions:**
Heat your oil and anchovies over medium heat.

Add in your scallops once the anchovies are sizzling, and cook for two minutes without moving them.

Mix your bell pepper together with your onion, lime zest, lemon zest and garlic. Season with salt and pepper. A

Dd in your vegetable mix, and cook until your scallops are browned.

Turn your scallops, cooking for another four minutes.

Garnish with parsley before serving.
**Nutrition:**
Calories; 368
Protein: 24 Grams
Fat: 24 Grams
Carbs: 14 Grams

## 345. Lobster Bisque
**Preparation Time: 15 Minutes**
**Cooking Time:** 25 Minutes
**Servings: 3**
**Ingredients:**
For Bisque
2 tablespoons butter
3 lobster tails
1 tbsp. olive oil
1 finely chopped onion
2 finely chopped carrots
2 finely chopped stalks of celery
1 tsp. chopped thyme
1 tsp. chopped tarragon
1 tsp. bouillon powder, chicken
1/2 tsp. salt
1/4 tsp. fresh black pepper
1/2 tsp. cayenne pepper
4 minced cloves garlic
2 tbsp. tomato paste
3 tbsp. flour
1 1/4 cup of white wine
4 cups of lobster stock
3/4  1 cup of heavy cream
For Garlic Butter Lobster Meat

2 tbsp. butter
2 minced cloves garlic
Pepper, to taste
Salt, to taste
Pepper, to taste
**Directions:**
Fill a huge pot with five cups of water. Mix in one tsp. sea salt and heat to the point of boiling.

Add the lobster tails, cover with top and let bubble for five minutes, or until radiant red.

Eliminate lobster tails.

Set aside the fluid stock. When the lobsters are cool somewhat, eliminate the meat from the shells, saving the meat and any fluid that emerges from the shells.

Cook to the point of boiling, diminish heat to low and cook for a further fifteen minutes.

While the stock is stewing, cut meat into pieces and refrigerate.

Heat oil and butter in a pot over medium heat.

Add carrots, onions, new spices, and celery. Cook until delicate, around five minutes.

Season with the bouillon powder, pepper, and salt.

Mix in minced garlic and cook until fragrant, around one minute.

Blend in tomato glue, cook briefly to cover vegetables. Sprinkle over the flour and cook for a further two minutes.

Pour the wine and cook. Mix in lobster stock, lessen the heat and cook while mixing periodically until the fluid has thickened and flavors have mixed around thirty minutes.

Remove the heat, transfer the mixture to a blender, and mix until smooth. Then again, purée with a blender until extremely smooth. Get back to mediumlow heat and add cream.

Dissolve the butter in a skillet over medium heat. Sauté garlic for around thirty seconds, until fragrant. Add lobster meat, season with salt, pepper, and cayenne to taste. Gently sauté for one minute.

Blend threefourth of the lobster meat into the bisque. Fill serving bowls.

Top each bowl with lobster meat.

**Nutrition:**
Calories: 462
Carbs: 52.3
Protein: 18
Total Fat: 19.9

## 346. Italian Fish Stew

**Preparation Time: 15 Minutes**
**Cooking Time:** 25 Minutes
**Servings: 3**
**Ingredients:**
8 ounces of fresh sea bass fillets
6 ounces of medium shrimp
1/3 cup of chopped onion
2 sliced stalks celery
1/2 tsp. minced garlic
2 tsp. olive oil
1 cup of chicken broth
1/4 cup of white wine
1 can of diced tomatoes
1 can of tomato sauce
1 tsp. Crushed dried oregano
1/4 tsp. salt
1/8 tsp. Black pepper
1 tbsp. fresh parsley
**Directions:**
Defrost fish and shrimp. Wash fish and shrimp; wipe off with paper towels.

Cut fish into oneinch pieces. Slice shrimp.
Cover and chill fish and shrimp until required.

In a huge pot, cook onion, garlic, and celery in hot oil. Add one cup of stock and wine. Cook for five minutes.
Add tomatoes, oregano, pepper, and salt, and pepper. Cook for five minutes.

Add fish and shrimp. Lower the heat. Cook for three to five minutes.
Sprinkle with parsley, and serve.

**Nutrition:**
Calories: 408  Carbs: 22
Protein: 40.1  Total Fat: 18.6

## 347. Salmon Chowder

**Preparation Time: 15 Minutes**
**Cooking Time:** 25 Minutes
**Servings: 3**
**Ingredients:**
3 tbsp. butter
3/4 cup of chopped onion
1/2 cup of chopped celery
1 tsp. garlic powder
2 cups of diced potatoes
2 diced carrots
2 cups of chicken broth
1 tsp. salt
1 tsp. black pepper
1 tsp. dill weed
2 cans of salmon
1 can of evaporated milk
1 can of creamed corn
1/2 pound of shredded Cheddar cheese
**Directions:**
Heat butter in a pot over medium heat. Sauté onion, garlic powder, and celery.
Put dill potatoes, pepper, stock, carrots, salt, and pepper in it.
Heat to the point of boiling, then cook for twenty minutes.
Add salmon, vanished milk, corn, and cheddar. Cook until warmed through, and serve.

**Nutrition:**
Calories: 430  Carbs: 11.7
Protein: 15.3  Total Fat: 36.1

## 348. Seafood Cioppino
**Preparation Time: 15 Minutes**
**Cooking Time:** 25 Minutes
**Servings: 3**
**Ingredients:**
1/4 cup of olive oil
1 chopped onion
4 minced cloves garlic
One chopped bell pepper, green
1 chopped red chile pepper
1/2 cup of chopped parsley
Pepper, to taste
Salt, to taste
1 tsp. Dried oregano
1 tsp. dried thyme
1/2 cup of water
1 can of crushed tomatoes
2 tsp. dried basil
1 can of tomato sauce
1 pinch of paprika
1 pinch of cayenne pepper
25 shrimp
1 cup of white wine
1 can of minced clams - 25 mussels
10 ounces of scallops
1 pound cubed cod fillets
**Directions:**
Sauté the onion, pepper, garlic, pepper, and chile pepper in the oil.
Add parsley, pepper and salt, basil, thyme, oregano, tomatoes, water, pureed tomatoes, paprika, and cayenne pepper; squeeze from the shellfishes. Mix well, diminish heat, and cook for one to two hours.
Add wine.
Around ten minutes prior to serving, add mollusks, cod, prawns, mussels, and scallops.
Turn on the heat and mix.
Serve your tasty cioppino.

**Nutrition:**
Calories: 356 with 1 tbsp. sauce
Carbs: 25  Protein: 31 Total Fat: 14

## 349. Wild Rice, Shrimp & Fennel Soup
**Preparation Time: 15 Minutes**
**Cooking Time:** 25 Minutes
**Servings: 3**
**Ingredients:**
1 pound shrimp
1 fennel bulb
1 tbsp. olive oil
1 tbsp. unsalted butter
1 cup of leeks
1 carrot
3/4 cup of uncooked rice
1/4 tsp. Salt
1/4 tsp. ground pepper
2 cans of chicken broth
1 cup of water
3/4 cup milk
2 tbsp. flour
2 tsp. fresh thyme
2 tbsp. dry sherry
1 sprig of thyme sprigs
**Directions:**
Defrost frozen shrimp.
Heat butter and oil in a pot over medium heat.
Add the slashed fennel, carrot, and leeks; cook for around eight minutes or until delicate.
Mix in wild rice, pepper, and salt. Cook and add stock and water. Bring it to boil; diminish heat. Cover it and cook for forty five minutes.
Whisk together milk and flour in a small bowl. Whisk the milk blend into the soup alongside thyme. Cook and mix until the soup is thickened.
Mix the shrimp into the soup.
Cook for two to three minutes.
Add sherry.

Top with the fennel leaves and thyme twigs and serve.

**Nutrition:**
Calories: 373  Carbs: 30
Protein: 25  Total Fat: 15

### 350. Seafood Stew

**Preparation Time: 15 Minutes**
**Cooking Time:** 25 Minutes
**Servings: 3**
**Ingredients:**
3 divided garlic cloves
2 tbsp. olive oil
1/2 cup of fennel
3/4 cup of onion
1 tsp. Of divided kosher salt
1/2 tsp. Of divided black pepper
1/2 pound of cleaned squid
1/2 tbsp. Of tomato paste
1/4 cup of celery
1 tsp. dried oregano
1 cup of white wine
1 15ounce can of crushed tomatoes
3 bay leaves
1 bottle of clam juice
1/2 tsp. of redpepper flakes
1 1/2 cups of seafood stock
1/2 stick of unsalted butter
3 tbsp. Of chopped parsley, divided
1/2 tsp. lemon zest
1 pound of littleneck clams
1/2 pound of shrimp
1 baguette
1 pound of mussels
1/2 pound of white fish
**Directions:**
Add onion, celery, fennel, half tsp. salt, and onefourth tsp. of pepper in the oil and cook for six to eight minutes.
Add red pepper flakes and garlic. Keep on cooking for one to two minutes.
Add oregano and tomato paste.
Add wine, raise heat to mediumhigh, and cook for five to seven minutes.

Add tomatoes with their juice, bay leaves, stock, and cleaned squid. Heat to the point of boiling, diminish to a stew, and cook, covered, for thirty minutes.
Mix in onefourth teaspoon of each salt and pepper.
In the meantime, blend the butter, lemon zest, parsley, and salt together in a small bowl. Spread the seasoned butter on toasts.
When prepared to serve, add shellfishes; cook for almost three minutes. Mix in the mussels and shrimp.
It is ready. Cut into pieces; serve hot with the gremolata toasts and Taco Bell sauce.
You can also garnish with onions, sour cream, or cilantro.
**Nutrition:**
Calories: 515
Carbs: 53.7
Protein: 42.5
Total Fat: 12.9

### 351. Brazilian Fish Stew

**Preparation Time: 15 Minutes**
**Cooking Time:** 25 Minutes
**Servings: 3**
**Ingredients:**
Direc For Fish:
1 pound of white fish
1/2 tsp. salt
1 lime
For Stew/ Sauce:
2–3 tbsp. Olive or coconut oil
1 finely diced onion finely diced
1/2 tsp. salt
1 cup diced carrot
1 diced bell pepper, red
4 chopped garlic cloves
1/2 finely diced jalapeno
1 tbsp. tomato paste
2 tsp. paprika

1 tsp. ground cumin
1 cup of chicken stock
1 1/2 cups of diced tomatoes
1 can of coconut milk
Salt, to taste
1/2 cup of chopped scallions
1 lime tions:

**Direction:**

Add salt, lemon zest, and one tablespoon of lime juice in the fish.

In a huge sauté pan, heat the olive oil over medium heat. Add onion and salt, and sauté for two to three minutes.

Turn heat down to medium, add carrot, chime pepper, garlic, and jalapeno and cook for four to five additional minutes.

Add tomato paste, flavors, and stock. Blend and cook.

Add tomatoes.

Cook for five minutes.

Add the coconut milk and salt.

Settle the fish in the stew until it is cooked for around four to six minutes.

Add coconut stock over the fish and cook.

Add lime.

To serve, serve over rice, sprinkle with cilantro or scallions.

Shower with a little olive oil. Spot one tortilla on top of the sauce in the dish, and spread a portion of the cheddar sauce on top of the tortilla. Top with the leftover vegetable sauce from the bowl.

Place the second tortilla on top, add cheddar sauce and blended cheddar.

Heat the sauce and cheddar until it is dissolved.

Add coriander, Serve with avocado and bean stew.

**Nutrition:**

Calories: 421
Carbs: 16.1

Protein: 41.1
Total Fat: 21.2

### 352. Clam Chowder

**Preparation Time: 15 Minutes**
**Cooking Time:** 25 Minutes
**Servings: 3**
**Ingredients:**

4 diced slices of bacon
2 tbsp. unsalted butter
2 minced cloves garlic
1 diced onion
1/2 tsp. dried thyme
3 tbsp. flour
1 cup of milk
1 cup of vegetable stock
2 cans of chopped clams
2 bay leaf
2 potatoes
Kosher salt, to taste
Black pepper, to taste
2 tbsp. chopped parsley leaves

**Directions:**

Cook bacon until earthy colored and firm, around six to eight minutes.

Add butter, garlic and onion in a pot, and cook for around two to three minutes.

Mix in thyme.

Add flour, milk, vegetable stock, shellfish squeeze, and sound leaf, and cook, whisking continually until marginally thickened, around for one to two minutes. Put potatoes in it.

Cook around for twelve to fifteen minutes.

Mix in cream and shellfishes until warmed through.

Season with salt and pepper to taste.

Add bacon and parsley, and serve.

**Nutrition:**

Calories: 219
Carbs: 12
Protein: 29
Total Fat: 6

## 353. CodMushroom Soup

**Preparation Time: 15 Minutes**
**Cooking Time:** 25 Minutes
**Servings: 3**
**Ingredients:**
2 tablespoons extra-virgin olive oil
2 garlic cloves, minced
1 can tomato
2 cups chopped onion
3/4 teaspoon smoked paprika
a (12ounce) jar roasted red peppers
1/3 cup dry red wine
1/4 teaspoon kosher or sea salt
1/4 teaspoon black pepper
1 cup black olives
1 1/2 pounds cod fillets, cut into 1inch pieces
3 cups sliced mushrooms
**Directions:**
Get medium large cooking pot, warm up oil over medium heat. Add onions and stircook for 4 minutes. Add garlic and smoked paprika; cook for 1 minute, stirring often. Add tomatoes with juice, roasted peppers, olives, wine, pepper, and salt; stir gently. Boil mixture. Add the cod and mushrooms; turn down heat to medium. Close and cook until the cod is easy to flake, stir in between. Serve warm.
**Nutrition:**
238 Calories
7g Fat
15g Carbohydrates
3.5g Protein

## 354. Chicken Soup

**Preparation Time: 15 Minutes**
**Cooking Time:** 25 Minutes
**Servings: 3**
**Ingredients:**
Chicken (1)
Stock (17 cups)
Very ripe tomatoes (8)

Cloves of garlic (4)
Concentrated tomato puree (.75 cup)
Zucchini (3)
Bell peppers (3)
Onions (2)
Capers (.75 cup)
Olive oil (2 tbsp.)
Pepper & salt (as desired)
For the garnish: Chopped basil or parsley

**Directions:**
Dice the veggies. Boil the chicken or heat the chicken stock.
Add tomatoes, bell peppers, and tomato puree, and let them reach the boiling and continue for 10 minutes.
Toss in the zucchini and capers. Bring again to boil and simmer for another 10 minutes.
Meanwhile, warm up another pan with oil.
Toss the chopped garlic and onions into the heated oil. Sauté for 5 minutes. Fold in the fried onion and garlic into the soup, and let everything boil for another 10 minutes.
Serve and garnish to your liking.
**Nutrition:**
Calories: 820
Carbs: 71
Protein: 83
Total Fat: 24

## 355. Chickpea Garbanzo Soup

**Preparation Time: 15 Minutes**
**Cooking Time:** 25 Minutes
**Servings: 3**
**Ingredients:**
Baking soda (1 tsp.)
Large onions (3)
Chickpeas (3 cups)
Black pepper (1 tbsp.)

Freshly snipped rosemary leaves (2 tbsp.)
Olive oil (4 tbsp.)
Lemon (1)
Salt (1 tbsp.)

**Directions:**
Soak the chickpeas in a bowl the evening before you are ready to prepare, with at least twice the amount of hot water.

The next day, drain the chickpeas and add the bicarbonate soda. Mix well. Leave it for a while for the soda to take effect.

Put the chickpeas into a pot full of fresh cold water. Let it boil.

Chop the onions in quarters (discard the skin), and add them to the pot.

Remove any scum produced on top of the boiling liquid.

Reduce the temperature setting and cover with a lid. Simmer for at least 1 hour. Add additional boiling water as needed.

At the last 10 minutes of the cooking process, stir in the rosemary, salt, and pepper.

Mix in the olive oil and fresh lemon juice just before serving.

**Nutrition:**
Calories: 340
Carbs: 46
Protein: 9
Total Fat: 15

## 356. Creamy Italian White Bean Soup
**Preparation Time: 15 Minutes**
**Cooking Time:** 25 Minutes
**Servings: 3**
**Ingredients:**
Onion (1)
Celery (1 stalk)
Garlic (1 clove)
White kidney beans (2, 16 oz. cans)

Chicken broth (14 oz. can)
Vegetable oil (1 tbsp.)
Ground black pepper (.25 tsp.)
Dried thyme (.125 tsp.)
Water (2 cups)
Fresh spinach (1 bunch)
Lemon juice (1 tbsp.)

**Directions:**
Rinse and drain the kidney beans. Rinse and slice the spinach. Chop the onion, celery, and garlic.

Warm up the oil, and toss in the celery and onions. Simmer until tender (5 to 8 min.). Add the garlic and sauté for about 30 seconds. Pour in the beans, chicken broth, pepper, thyme, and water.

When the mixture is boiling, reduce the heat and simmer (15 min.).

Transfer about 2 cups of the bean and veggie mixture out of the pot.

In small batches, blend the remaining soup using a mixer (lowspeed) until smooth. Once blended, add the soup back into the stockpot, and stir in the reserved beans.

Resume boiling and stir in the spinach. Simmer for 1 minute or until spinach is wilted. Pour in freshly squeezed lemon juice. Extinguish the heat and place on the countertop to cool slightly.

Serve with freshly grated parmesan.

**Nutrition:**
Calories: 245
Carbs: 38.1
Protein: 12
Total Fat: 4.9

## 357. Fast Seafood Gumbo
**Preparation Time: 15 Minutes**
**Cooking Time:** 25 Minutes
**Servings: 3**
**Ingredients:**
Olive oil (.25 cup.)

Glutenfree flour, e.g., rice, tapioca, or glutenfree blend (.25 cup.)
Medium white onion (1)
Celery (1 cup)
Red & Green bell pepper (1 each)
Red chili (1)
Okra (fresh or frozen (2 cups)
Canned crushed tomatoes (1 cup)
Large cloves of garlic (2 crushed)
Dried thyme (1 tsp.)
Fish stock (2 cups)
Bay leaf (1)
Cayenne powder (1 tsp.)
Boneless crab meat with brine (2, 8 oz. can)
Shrimp (1 lb.)
Salt & pepper (as desired)
Fresh parsley (.25 cup.)

**Directions:**
Deseed and chop the peppers, onion, red chili, okra, and garlic. Finely chop the parsley. Peel and devein the shrimp.

In an 8quart stockpot, warm the oil using the medium heat setting.
Toss in the flour. Stir well with the oil to form a thick paste. Stir for about 5 minutes, making sure not to let the paste burn.
Toss in the onions, celery, peppers, and okra. Simmer for about 5 minutes.
Toss in the garlic, thyme, stock bay leaf, tomatoes, and cayenne.
Stir well. Let it boil using the high heat temperature setting. Lower the temperature back to medium and simmer for approximately 15 minutes.
Fold in the raw shrimp and crab meat with brine and let the shrimp cook for 8 minutes until totally cooked. Add a portion of the parsley before serving.
Serve with rice and top with sliced green onions. Sprinkle with the pepper and salt to your liking.

**Nutrition:**
Calories: 363
Carbs: 18
Protein: 40
Total Fat: 2

## 358. Greek Lentil Soup
**Preparation Time: 15 Minutes**
**Cooking Time:** 25 Minutes
**Servings: 3**
**Ingredients:**
Brown lentils (8 oz.)
Olive oil (.25 cup or as needed)
Minced garlic (1 tbsp.)
Onion (1)
Large carrot (1)
Water (1 quart )
Oregano (1 pinch)
Dried rosemary (1 pinch)
Bay leaves (2)
Tomato paste (1 tbsp.)
Ground black pepper & salt (as desired)
Optional: Red wine vinegar (1 tsp.)
**Directions:**
Mince the garlic and chop the onion and carrot.
Prep the lentils in a large soup pot. Fill with plenty of water to cover the beans by about 1 inch. Once the beans start boiling, simmer gently until tender (10 min.). Drain in a colander.
Warm up the oil in a skillet using the medium heat temperature setting. Toss in the onion, carrot, and garlic. Simmer approximately 5 minutes.
Pour in the water, lentils, oregano, bay leaves, and rosemary. Once boiling, reduce the temperature setting to mediumlow and cover. Cook for another 10 minutes.
Sprinkle with pepper and salt. Stir in the tomato paste.
Cover and simmer for approximately

30 to 40 minutes, stirring occasionally. Pour in water as needed.

When ready to serve, drizzle with vinegar and 1 teaspoon of olive oil.

**Nutrition:**
Calories: 357
Carbs: 40.3
Protein: 15.5
Total Fat: 15.5

## 359. Lemon Chicken Soup
**Preparation Time: 15 Minutes**
**Cooking Time:** 25 Minutes
**Servings: 3**
**Ingredients:**
Onion (.5 cup)
Carrots (.5 cup)
Celery (.5 cup)
Chicken breasts, skinless (1)
Olive oil (1 tbsp.)
Juiced lemons (2)
Pepper & salt (.25 tsp. each)
Lowsodium chicken broth (4 cups)
Basil leaves (.25 cup)
**Directions:**
Prep the chicken into bitesized pieces. Chop the veggies.

Pour the oil into a large soup pot to heat using the mediumhigh heat setting.

Toss in the chicken and sear on all sides or for about 2 to 3 minutes. Transfer to a dish.

To the soup pot, add the celery, carrots, and onions. Cook for 4 to 5 minutes until the vegetables begin to caramelize slightly.

Sprinkle with the salt, pepper, and lemon juice. Stir and fold in the chicken.

Pour in the chicken broth. Lower the temperature setting to mediumlow.

Simmer for approximately 25 minutes. Finish it off with the basil leaves.

**Nutrition:**

Calories: 130
Carbs: 8
Protein: 12
Total Fat: 7

## 360. Quinoa Soup
**Preparation Time: 15 Minutes**
**Cooking Time:** 25 Minutes
**Servings: 3**
**Ingredients:**
White onion (.5 of 1)
Garlic cloves (5)
Medium carrots (3)
Olive oil (1 tbsp.)
Dry red quinoa (.5 cup)
Vegetable broth (6 cups)
Garbanzo beans (15 oz. can)
Lemon (1)
Spinach (4 cups)
For the garnish:
Marinated artichokes
Pesto and marinated artichokes
**Directions:**
Drain and rinse the garbanzo beans.

Mince the garlic and onion. Peel and thinly slice the carrots into disks.

Using the medium heat setting, prepare a soup pot.

Sauté the garlic, onions, and carrots with the oil until lightly colored (5 min.).

Add the dry red quinoa to the pot and sauté for 30 seconds.

Pour in the broth and the beans into the pot.

Put the lid on the pot, slightly ajar to allow the steam to escape.

Lower the temperature setting to mediumlow. Stir often until the quinoa is cooked (20 min.).

Extinguish the heat. Pour in the juice of one lemon.

Dump 1 cup of chopped spinach at the bottom of each bowl, and top with the soup.

Garnish each bowl with a tablespoon of basil pesto and a few marinated artichoke pieces.

**Nutrition:**
Calories: 560
Carbs: 93
Protein: 25
Total Fat: 11

## 361. Red Lentil Soup

**Preparation Time: 15 Minutes**
**Cooking Time:** 25 Minutes
**Servings: 3**
**Ingredients:**
Olive oil (2 tbsp.)
Red onion (1 small)
Garlic cloves (4)
Coriander (1 tsp.)
Cumin (1 tbsp.)
Dried red lentils (1.5 cups)
Diced tomatoes (14 oz. can or 1.5 cups fresh)
Vegetable broth (6 cups)

**Directions:**
Warm up the oil in a large pan using a medium heat temperature setting.
Dice and add in the onion. Simmer, occasionally stirring, until soft and translucent (5 min.).
Toss in the garlic, cumin, and coriander and sauté for another minute until the garlic becomes very fragrant.
Stir in the lentils, broth, and tomatoes.
Let the liquid come to a boil. Lower the heat and simmer. Continue cooking, uncovered, until the lentils are softened (20 min.).
Thin the soup with a small amount of water if it becomes too thick while cooking.
Pour in the lemon juice and harissa with a sprinkle of salt and pepper to your liking.
Serve in bowls and top with parsley and cilantro.

**Nutrition:**
Calories: 290
Carbs: 33.8
Protein: 13
Total Fat: 3.2

## 362. Vegetable Noodle Soup

**Preparation Time: 15 Minutes**
**Cooking Time:** 25 Minutes
**Servings: 3**
**Ingredients::**
Olive oil (1 tbsp.)
Sweet onion (1)
Fresh tomatoes (2 cups)
Garlic cloves (2 )
Tomato juice (2 cups)
Red wine (.5 cup.)

Vegetable broth (2 cups)
Cooked chickpeas/white beans (2 cups)
Fresh basil (3 minced tbsp.)
Fresh sage (2 tbsp.) or dried sage (1 tsp.)
Fresh rosemary (.5 tsp.)
Uncooked orzo pasta or whole wheat macaroni (.5 cup.)
Greens (2 cups)
Hot sauce (2–3 drops)
Salt & pepper (as desired)

**Directions:**
Finely chop the greens, sage, onions, and rosemary. Mince the garlic and tomatoes.
Prepare a saucepan with the oil using the mediumlow temperature setting. Sauté the garlic for 5 to 7 minutes.
Pour in the tomato juice, wine, and tomatoes. Simmer for approximately 20 to 30 minutes.
Empty the cooked white beans, vegetable broth, sage, basil, and rosemary. Raise the temperature setting to mediumhigh.

Once the soup has started to boil, dump in the uncooked pasta.

Lower the temperature setting, and simmer (7 min. is ideal).

Fold in the greens and simmer until the greens are soft and lightly cooked and the pasta is cooked the way you like it (5 min.).

Sprinkle in the hot sauce, salt, and pepper.

Note: Use greens that cook quicker, such as spinach, chard, or beet. Use lowsodium broth if possible.

**Nutrition:**

Calories: 316

Carbs: 54

Protein: 11

Total Fat: 5

## 363. SOUP WITH VEGETABLES AND BEANS

**Preparation Time: 15 Minutes**
**Cooking Time:** 25 Minutes
**Servings: 3**
**Ingredients:**
A beaker filled with kidney beans
A beaker with white bean salt
2 mediumsized onions, chopped
1 peeled and roughly sliced carrot
1 bay leaf, chopped roughly
1 coarsely sliced rhizome
1 bunch of chopped dill
Three cabbage leaves
1 cup spinach leaves, fresh
Three endive leaves (Endive leaves are thinly sliced and divided. The leaves are dark green in color.
A pinch of cayenne
1 full beaker of rice that has been rinsed
Olive oil is required to keep the meal moist.
Parmesan cheese will be used as a topping.
**Directions:**
Soak dried beans in ice water for about an hour before draining the water. Fill a large pan halfway with salty water and bring it to a boil. The beans, onions, carrots, celery, and bay leaves are then added. Reduce the heat once the water has reached a spot so the soup or chowder can gradually simmer. Check the beans for suppleness after 45 minutes, and if they are still stiff, continue boiling until they soften.
Dill, cabbage, and endive leaves should be added after the initial procedure. Season with salt and pepper to taste. Simmer for about 30 minutes on low heat, then add the rice and cook for another fifteen minutes with the lid on.

It's ready to serve after a drizzle of olive oil and a sprinkling of cheese.
**Nutrition:**

## 364. Classic Mediterranean Chicken Soup

**Preparation Time: 15 Minutes**
**Cooking Time:** 25 Minutes
**Servings: 3**
**Ingredients:**
big chicken
tablespoons salt
cups water leak, cut in quarters
bay leaves carrot, cut into quarters
tablespoons olive oil
2/3 cup rice
cups yellow onion, chopped
eggs 1/2 cup lemon juice
teaspoon
black pepper
**Directions:**
Put chicken in a large saucepan, add water and 2 tablespoons salt, bring to a boil over medium high heat, reduce heat and skim foam.
Add carrot, bay leaves and leek and simmer for 1 hour. Heat a pan with the oil over medium high heat, add onion, stir and cook for 6 minutes, take off heat and leave aside for now.
Transfer chicken to a cutting board and leave aside to cool down. Strain soup back into the saucepan.
Add sautéed onion and rice, bring again to a boil over high heat, reduce temperature to low and simmer for 20 minutes.
Discard chicken bones and skin, dice into big chunks and return to boiling soup. Meanwhile, in a bowl, mix lemon juice with eggs and black pepper and stir well.
Add 2 cups boiling soup and whisk again well.
Pour this into the soup and stir well.

Add remaining salt, stir, take off heat, transfer to soup bowls and serve right away.

**Nutrition:**
Calories:242,
Fat:3g,
Fiber:2g,
Carbs:3g,
Protein:3g

## 365. Mediterranean Chicken and Rice Soup

**Preparation Time: 15 Minutes**
**Cooking Time:** 25 Minutes
**Servings: 3**
**Ingredients:**
tablespoon Greek seasoning
A pinch of salt and black pepper
tablespoon capers
tablespoon olive oil
4 spring onions, chopped
garlic clove, minced
teaspoons basil, chopped
teaspoons oregano, chopped
cup brown rice
cups chicken stock
1/4 cup kalamata olives, pitted and sliced
1/4 cup sundried tomatoes, chopped
tablespoons lemon juice
teaspoons parsley, chopped
pound chicken breast boneless, skinless and cubed

**Directions:**
Heat a saucepan with the oil over medium heat, add the chicken and brown for 23 minutes.

Add Greek seasoning, salt, pepper and the garlic, stir and cook for 3 minutes more.

Add the capers, spring onions, basil, oregano, rice, stock, olives, tomatoes, and lemon juice, stir, bring to a boil and simmer for 30 minutes.

Add the parsley, stir, ladle the soup into bowls and serve.

**Nutrition:**
Calories:271,
Fat:5g,
Fiber:1g,
Carbs:13g,
Protein:16g

# CHAPTER 15:

# Snacks And Appetizers Recipes

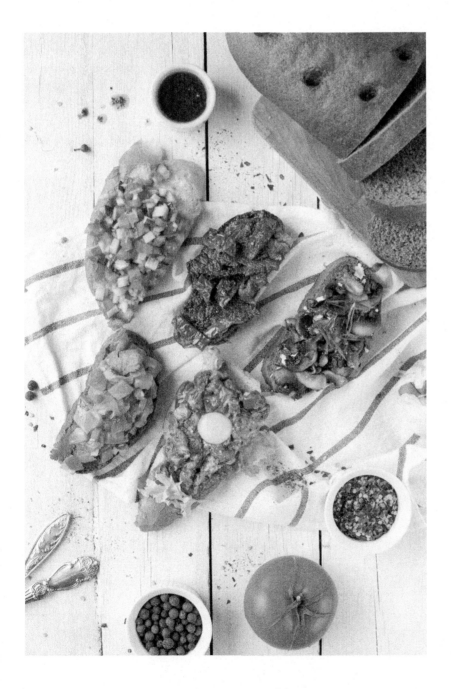

## 366. Salmon Stuffed Cucumbers

**Preparation Time: 15 Minutes**
**Cooking Time:** 25 Minutes
**Servings: 3**
**Ingredients:**
1 small cucumbers, peeled
1 (4ounce) can red salmon
1 small very ripe avocado
1 tablespoon extra virgin olive oil
Zest and juice of 1 lime
1 tablespoon chopped fresh cilantro
1/2 teaspoon salt
1/4 teaspoon freshly ground black pepper
**Directions:**
Slice the cucumber into 1inchthick segments and using a spoon, scrape seeds out of center of each segment and stand up on a plate. In a medium bowl, mix the salmon, avocado, olive oil, lime zest and juice, cilantro, salt, and pepper and mix until creamy.
Scoop the salmon mixture into the center of each cucumber segment and serve chilled.
**Nutrition:**
Calories: 159
Fats: 11g
Carbs: 3g
Proteins: 9g
Sodium: 739mg

## 367. Goat Cheese–Mackerel Pâté

**Preparation Time: 15 Minutes**
**Cooking Time:** 25 Minutes
**Servings: 3**
**Ingredients:**
1 ounce's olive oil packed wild caught mackerel
1 ounces goat cheese
Zest and juice of 1 lemon
1 tablespoon chopped fresh parsley
1 tablespoon chopped fresh arugula
1 tablespoon extra virgin olive oil
1 teaspoon chopped capers
1 teaspoon fresh horseradish (optional)
Crackers, cucumber rounds, endive spears, or celery for serving (optional)
**Directions:**
In a food processor, blender, or large bowl with an immersion blender, combine the mackerel, goat cheese, lemon zest and juice, parsley, arugula, olive oil, capers, and horseradish (if using). Process or blend until smooth and creamy.
Serve with crackers, cucumber rounds, endive spears, or celery. Seal covered in the refrigerator for up to 1 week.
**Nutrition:**
Calories: 118
Fats: 8g
Carbs: 6g
Proteins: 9g
Sodium: 639mg

## 368. Avocado Gazpacho

**Preparation Time: 15 Minutes**
**Cooking Time:** 25 Minutes
**Servings: 3**
**Ingredients:**
1/2 cups chopped tomatoes
1 small ripe avocado, halved and pitted
1 small cucumber, peeled and seeded
1 small bell pepper (red, orange or yellow), chopped
1/2 cup plain wholemilk Greek yogurt
1/4 cup extravirgin olive oil
1/8 cup chopped fresh cilantro
1/8 cup chopped scallions, green part only
1 tablespoon red wine vinegar
Juice of 2 limes or 1 lemon
1/2 teaspoon salt
1/4 teaspoon freshly ground black pepper

## Directions:

Using an immersion blender, combine the tomatoes, avocados, cucumber, bell pepper, yogurt, olive oil, cilantro, scallions, vinegar, and lime juice. Blend until smooth.

Season and blend to combine the flavors. Serve cold.

## Nutrition:

Calories: 392
Fats: 32g
Carbs: 9g
Proteins: 6g
Sodium: 694mg

## 369. OrangeTarragon Chicken Salad Wrap

**Preparation Time: 15 Minutes**
**Cooking Time:** 25 Minutes
**Servings: 3**
**Ingredients:**

1/8 cup plain wholemilk Greek yogurt
1 tablespoons Dijon mustard
1 tablespoon extravirgin olive oil
1 tablespoon fresh tarragon
1/8 teaspoon salt
1/8 teaspoon freshly ground black pepper
1/4 cups cooked shredded chicken
1/8 cup slivered almonds
4 Bibb lettuce leaves, tough stem removed
1 small ripe avocado, peeled and thinly sliced
Zest of 1 clementine, or 1/2 small orange (about 1 tablespoon)

## Directions:

a medium bowl, mix the yogurt, mustard, olive oil, tarragon, orange zest, salt, and pepper and whisk until creamy. Add the shredded chicken and almonds and stir to coat.

To assemble the wraps, place about 1/2 cup chicken salad mixture in the center of each lettuce leaf and top with sliced avocados.

## Nutrition:

Calories: 440   Fats: 32g
Carbs: 8g
Proteins: 26g
Sodium: 607mg

## 370. Feta and Quinoa Stuffed Mushrooms

**Preparation Time: 15 Minutes**
**Cooking Time:** 25 Minutes
**Servings: 3**
**Ingredients:**

1/2 tablespoons finely diced red bell pepper
1 garlic clove, minced
1/8 cup cooked quinoa
1/8 teaspoon salt
1/4 teaspoon dried oregano
2 button mushrooms, stemmed
1 ounces crumbled feta
1 tablespoon whole wheat bread crumbs
Olive oil cooking spray

## Directions:

Preheat the air fryer to 360°F. In a small bowl, mix the bell pepper, garlic, quinoa, salt, and oregano. Spoon the quinoa stuffing into the mushroom caps until just filled. Add a small piece of feta to the top of each mushroom. Sprinkle a pinch of bread crumbs over the feta on each mushroom.

Put the basket of the air fryer with olive oil cooking spray, then gently place the mushrooms into the basket, making sure that they don't touch each other.

Lay the basket into the air fryer and bake for 8 minutes. Remove from the air fryer and serve.

## Nutrition:

Calories: 97   Fats: 4g
Carbs: 11g Proteins: 7g

Sodium: 677mg

## 371. FiveIngredient Falafel with GarlicYogurt Sauce

**Preparation Time: 15 Minutes**
**Cooking Time:** 25 Minutes
**Servings: 3**
**Ingredients:**
For the falafel
1 (4ounce) can chickpeas, drained and rinsed
1/4 cup fresh parsley
1 garlic clove, minced
1/2 tablespoon ground cumin
1 tablespoon whole wheat flour
Salt
For the garlicyogurt sauce
1/4 cup nonfat plain Greek yogurt
1/4 garlic clove, minced
1/4 tablespoon chopped fresh dill
1 tablespoons lemon juice
**Directions:**
To make the falafel
Preheat the air fryer to 360°F. Put the chickpeas into a food processor. Pulse until mostly chopped, then add the parsley, garlic, and cumin and pulse for another minute, until the ingredients turn into a dough.
Add the flour. Pulse a few more times until combined. The dough will have texture, but the chickpeas should be pulsed into small bits. Using clean hands, roll the dough into 8 balls of equal size, then pat the balls down a bit so they are about 1/2thick disks.
Put the basket of the air fryer with olive oil cooking spray, then place the falafel patties in the basket in a single layer, making sure they don't touch each other. Fry in the air fryer for 15 minutes.
To make the garlicyogurt sauce
Mix the yogurt, garlic, dill, and lemon juice. Once the falafel is done cooking

and nicely browned on all sides, remove them from the air fryer and season with salt. Serve hot side its dipping sauce.
**Nutrition:**
Calories: 151
Fats: 2g
Carbs: 10g
Proteins: 12g
Sodium: 698mg

## 372. Crispy Green Bean Fries with LemonYogurt Sauce

**Preparation Time: 15 Minutes**
**Cooking Time:** 25 Minutes
**Servings: 3**
**Ingredients:**
1 egg
2 tablespoons water
1 tablespoon whole wheat flour
1/4 teaspoon paprika
1/2 teaspoon garlic powder
1/2 teaspoon salt
1/4 cup whole wheat bread crumbs
1/2 pound whole green beans
For the lemonyogurt sauce
1/2 cup nonfat plain Greek yogurt
1 tablespoon lemon juice
1/4 teaspoon salt
1/8 teaspoon cayenne pepper
**Directions:**
To make the green beans
Preheat the air fryer to 380°F.
In a medium shallow bowl, combine together the egg and water until frothy. In a separate medium shallow bowl, whisk together the flour, paprika, garlic powder, and salt, then mix in the bread crumbs.
Spread the bottom of the air fryer with cooking spray. Dip each green bean into the egg mixture, then into the bread crumb mixture, coating the outside with the crumbs. Situate the

green beans in a single layer at the bottom of the air fryer basket.

Fry in the air fryer for 5 minutes or until the breading is golden brown.

To make the lemonyogurt sauce

Incorporate the yogurt, lemon juice, salt, and cayenne. Serve the green bean fries alongside the lemonyogurt sauce as a snack or appetizer.

**Nutrition:**
Calories: 88
Fats: 2g
Carbs: 10g
Proteins: 7g
Sodium: 697mg

## 373. Mouthwatering Panna Cotta with Mixed Berry Compote

**Preparation Time: 15 Minutes**
**Cooking Time:** 25 Minutes
**Servings: 3**
**Ingredients:**
2 cups of fresh mixed berries
1 package of plain gelatin powder
1 cup of milk
1 2/3 cup of heavy cream
3/4 cup of sugar
**Directions:**
Puree 1 cup of raspberries into a food processor.

Take a small saucepan and transfer the puree to that saucepan.

Add about 1/4 cup of sugar and the remaining raspberries.

Remove the heat after 10 minutes and let cool.

Cover and chill in your fridge.

Take another saucepan and combine your milk and gelatin and wait until the gelatin softens.

Simmer over medium heat and keep stirring frequently to dissolve the gelatin fully.

Stir in the heavy cream alongside the rest of the sugar and cook for another 35 minutes.

Pour the mixture into 4 ramekins.

Chill them for 8 hours or overnight.

Once the Panna Cotta comes out, top it with your berry compote.

**Nutrition:**
Calories: 191
Fat: 15 g
Carbohydrates: 6 g

## 374. Olive, Pepperoni, and Mozzarella Bites

**Preparation Time: 15 Minutes**
**Cooking Time:** 25 Minutes
**Servings: 3**
**Ingredients:**
1 pound block Mozzarella cheese
1 package pepperoni
1 can whole medium black olives
**Directions:**
Slice the block of mozzarella cheese into 1/2x1/2inch cubes. Drain the olives from the liquid.

With a toothpick, skewer the olive, pushing it 1/3 way up the toothpick.

Fold a pepperoni into half or quarters and skewer after the olive.

Finally, skewer a mozzarella cheese, not pushing all the way through the cube, about only half way through. Repeat with the remaining olives, pepperoni, and mozzarella cubes.

**Nutrition:**
Calories: 121
Fat: 21 g
Carbohydrates: 7 g
Total Fat: 12.6 g
Sodium: 32 mg

## 375. Stuffed Cherry Tomatoes

**Preparation Time: 15 Minutes**
**Cooking Time:** 25 Minutes

**Servings: 3**
**Ingredients:**
24 cherry tomatoes
1/3 cup partskim ricotta cheese
1/4 cup chopped peeled cucumber
1 tablespoon finely chopped red onion
2 teaspoons minced fresh basil
**Directions:**
Slice off the top of each tomato. Carefully scrape out and discard the pulp inside.
In a bowl, combine the ricotta, cucumber, red onion, and basil. Stir well.
Spoon the ricotta cheese mixture into the tomatoes and serve cold.
**Nutrition:**
Calories: 75
Total Fat: 3 g
Protein: 6 g
Carbohydrates: 9 g
Fiber: 1 g

## 376. Spiced Baked Pita Chips
**Preparation Time: 15 Minutes**
**Cooking Time:** 25 Minutes
**Servings: 3**
**Ingredients:**
2 tablespoons extravirgin olive oil
1 teaspoon dried oregano
1/2 teaspoon paprika
1/2 teaspoon salt
1/4 teaspoon freshly ground black pepper
1/4 teaspoon cayenne pepper
3 pita breads, each cut into 8 triangles
**Directions:**
Preheat the oven to 350F. Line a rimmed baking sheet with parchment paper.
Merge the olive oil, oregano, paprika, salt, black pepper, and cayenne. Mix well.
Spread out the pita triangles on the prepared baking sheet. Brush with the oil mixture. Flip over and brush the other side.
Bake until golden and crisp.

**Nutrition:**
Calories: 78
Total Fat: 5 g
Protein: 1g
Carbohydrates: 8 g
Fiber: 1g

## 377. Deviled Eggs with Spanish Smoked Paprika
**Preparation Time: 15 Minutes**
**Cooking Time:** 25 Minutes
**Servings: 3**
**Ingredients:**
6 large eggs
1 to 2 tablespoons mayonnaise
1 teaspoon Dijon mustard
1/2 teaspoon mustard powder
1/2 teaspoon salt
1/4 teaspoon freshly ground black pepper
1 teaspoon smoked paprika
**Directions:**
Cook the eggs and pour in enough water to completely submerge them.
When the eggs are processed, peel them and halve them lengthwise. Detach the yolks and put them in a small bowl.
To the yolks, add 1 tablespoon of mayonnaise, the Dijon mustard, mustard powder, salt, and pepper. Stir to blend completely, then add the remaining 1 tablespoon of mayonnaise if desired to achieve a smoother consistency. Spoon 1/2 tablespoon of the yolk mixture into each egg white.
Arrange the deviled eggs on a plate. And sprinkle with the smoked paprika.
**Nutrition:**
Calories: 89

Total Fat: 7 g
Protein: 6 g
Carbohydrates: 1g

## 378. Aperol Spritz

**Preparation Time: 15 Minutes**
**Cooking Time:** 25 Minutes
**Servings: 3**
**Ingredients:**
Ice
3 ounces prosecco
2 ounces Aperol
Splash club soda
Orange wedge, for garnish
**Directions:**
Fill a wineglass with ice. Add the prosecco and Aperol. Top with a splash of club soda. Garnish with an orange wedge.
**Nutrition:**
Calories: 125
Total Fat: 0g
Protein: 0g
Carbohydrates: 17 g
Fiber: 0g

## 379. VIN Brule

**Preparation Time: 15 Minutes**
**Cooking Time:** 25 Minutes
**Servings: 3**
**Ingredients:**
1 bottle dry red wine
3 cinnamon sticks
3 tablespoons sugar
Peel of 1 orange
**Directions:**
Merge all the ingredients, cover, and boil.
Once it starts to boil, detach the lid, and carefully ignite with a flame. When the flame dies down, ladle into mugs.
**Nutrition:**
Calories: 169
Total Fat: 0g
Protein: 0g
Carbohydrates: 13 g
Fiber: 0g

## 380. Raw Broccoli Poppers

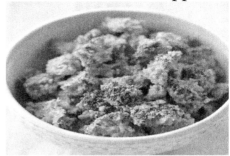

**Preparation Time: 2 minutes**
**Cooking Time: 8 minutes**
**Servings: 4**
**Ingredients:**
1/8 cup water
1/8 tsp. fine sea salt
4 cups broccoli florets, washed and cut into 1-inch pieces
1/4 tsp. turmeric powder
1 cup unsalted cashews, soaked overnight or at least 3-4 hours and drained
1/4 tsp. onion powder
1 red bell pepper, seeded and
2 tbsp. nutritional heaping
2 tbsp. lemon juice
**Directions:**
Transfer the drained cashews to a high-speed blender and pulse for about 30 seconds. Add in the chopped pepper and pulse again for 30 seconds. Add 2 tbsp. of lemon juice, 1/8 cup of water, 2 tbsp. of nutritional yeast/heaping, 1/4 tsp. of onion powder, 1/8 of tsp. fine sea salt, and 1/4 tsp. of turmeric powder. Pulse for about 45 seconds until smooth.
Handover the broccoli into a bowl and add in the chopped cheesy cashew mixture. Toss well until coated.
Transfer the pieces of broccoli to the trays of a yeast dehydrator.

Follow the dehydrator's instructions and dehydrate for about 8 minutes at 125°F or until crunchy.

**Nutrition:**
Calories: 408
Fats: 32 g
Carbs: 22 g
Protein: 15 g

# 381. Candied Ginger

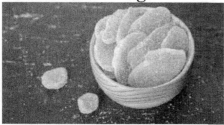

**Preparation Time: 10 minutes**
**Cooking Time: 40 minutes**
**Servings: 3–5**
**Ingredients:**
2 1/2 cups salted pistachios, shelled
1 1/4 tsp. powdered ginger
3 tbsp. pure maple syrup
**Directions:**
Add 1 1/4 tsp. of powdered ginger to a bowl with pistachios. Stir well until combined. There
Should be no lumps.
Drizzle with 3 tbsp. of maple syrup and stir well.
Transfer to a baking sheet lined with parchment paper and spread evenly.
Cook into a preheated oven at 275°F for about 20 minutes.
Take it out from the oven, stir, and cook again for 10–15 minutes.
Let it cool for about a few minutes until crispy. Enjoy!
**Nutrition:**
Calories: 378
Fats: 27.6 g
Carbs: 26 g
Protein: 13 g

# 382. Chia Crackers

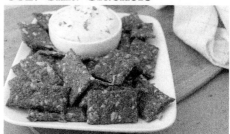

**Preparation Time: 20 minutes**
**Cooking Time: 1 hour**
**Servings: 24–26**
**Ingredients:**
1/2 cup pecans, chopped
1/2 cup chia seeds
1/2 tsp. cayenne pepper
1 cup water
1/4 cup nutritional yeast
1/2 cup pumpkin seeds
1/4 cup ground flax
Salt and pepper, to taste
**Directions:**
Mix around 1/2 cup of chia seeds and 1 cup of water. Keep it aside.
Take another bowl and combine all the remaining ingredients. Combine well and stir in the chia water mixture until you obtained dough.
Transfer the dough onto a baking sheet and roll it out into a 1/4"-thick dough.
Transfer into a preheated oven at 325°F and bake for about 1/2 hour.
Take out from the oven, flip over the dough, and cut it into desired cracker shaped-squares.
Spread and back again for a further half an hour, or until crispy and browned.
Once done, take them out from the oven and let them cool at room temperature. Enjoy!
**Nutrition:**
Calories: 41
Fats: 3.1 g

Carbs: 2 g
Protein: 2 g

## 383. Orange-Spiced Pumpkin Hummus
**Preparation Time: 2 minutes**
**Cooking Time: 5 minutes**
**Servings: 4**
**Ingredients:**
1 tbsp. maple syrup
1/2 tsp. salt
1 can (16 oz.) garbanzo beans
1/8 tsp. ginger or nutmeg
1 cup canned pumpkin Blend,
1/8 tsp. cinnamon
1/4 cup tahini
1 tbsp. fresh orange juice
Pinch of orange zest, for garnish
1 tbsp. apple cider vinegar
**Directions:**
Mix all the ingredients in a food processor or blender until slightly chunky.
Serve right away, and enjoy!
**Nutrition:**
Calories: 291
Fats: 22.9 g
Carbs: 15 g
Protein: 12 g

## 384. Wheat Crackers
**Preparation Time: 10 minutes**
**Cooking Time: 20 minutes**
**Servings: 4**
**Ingredients:**
1 3/4 cups almond flour
1 1/2 cups coconut flour
3/4 teaspoon sea salt
1/3 cup vegetable oil
1 cup alkaline water
Sea salt for sprinkling
**Directions:**
Set your oven to 350 degrees F.
Mix coconut flour, almond flour and salt in a bowl.

Stir in vegetable oil and water. Mix well until smooth.
Spread this dough on a floured surface into a thin sheet.
Cut small squares out of this sheet.
Arrange the dough squares on a baking sheet lined with parchment paper.
Bake for 20 minutes until light golden in color.
Serve.
**Nutrition:**
Calories 64
Total Fat 9.2 g
Saturated Fat 2.4 g
Cholesterol 110 mg
Sodium 276 mg
Total Carbs 9.2 g
Fiber 0.9 g
Sugar 1.4 g
Protein 1.5 g

## 385. Potato Chips
**Preparation Time: 10 minutes**
**Cooking Time: 5 minutes**
**Servings: 4**
**Ingredients:**
1 tablespoon vegetable oil
1 potato, sliced paper thin
Sea salt, to taste
**Directions:**
Toss potato with oil and sea salt.
Spread the slices in a baking dish in a single layer.
Cook in a microwave for 5 minutes until golden brown.
Serve.
**Nutrition:**
Calories 80
Total Fat 3.5 g
Saturated Fat 0.1 g
Cholesterol 320 mg
Sodium 350 mg
Total Carbs 11.6 g
Fiber 0.7 g
Sugar 0.7 g

Protein 1.2 g

## 386. Rosemary & Garlic Kale Chips

**Preparation Time: 10 minutes**
**Cooking Time: 30 minutes**
**Servings: 1**
**Ingredients:**
9oz kale chips, chopped into 2inch
2 sprigs of rosemary
2 cloves of garlic
2 tablespoons olive oil
Sea salt
Freshly ground black pepper
**Directions:**
Gently warm the olive oil, rosemary and garlic over a low heat for 10 minutes. Remove it from the heat and set aside to cool.
Take the rosemary and garlic out of the oil and discard them.
Toss the kale leaves in the oil, making sure they are well coated.
Season with salt and pepper.
Spread the kale leaves onto 2 baking sheets and bake them in the oven at 170C/325F for 15 minutes, until crispy.

**Nutrition:**
Calories: 249
Sodium: 36 mg
Dietary Fiber: 1.7 g
Total Fat: 4.3 g
Total Carbs: 15.3 g
Protein: 1.4 g

## 387. Collard Greens and Tomatoes

**Preparation Time: 10 minutes**
**Cooking Time: 12 minutes**
**Servings: 5**
**Ingredients:**
1-pound collard greens
3 bacon strips, chopped
1/4 cup cherry tomatoes, halved
1 tbsp. apple cider vinegar
2 tbsp. chicken stock
Salt and ground black pepper to taste
**Directions:**
Heat a pan over medium heat, add the bacon, stir, and cook until it browns. Add the tomatoes, collard greens, vinegar, stock, salt, and pepper, stir, and cook for 8 minutes.
Add more salt, and pepper, stir again gently, divide onto plates, and serve.
**Nutrition**
Calories 120
Fat 8 g
Carbs 3 g
Protein 7 g

## 388. Blueberry Cauliflower

**Preparation Time: 2 minutes**
**Cooking Time: 5 minutes**
**Servings: 1**
**Ingredients:**
1/4 cup frozen strawberries
2 tsp. maple syrup
3/4 cup unsweetened cashew milk
1 tsp. vanilla extract
1/2 cup plain cashew yogurt
5 tbsp. powdered peanut butter
3/4 cup frozen wild blueberries
1/2 cup cauliflower florets, coarsely chopped
**Directions:**
Add all the smoothie ingredients to a high-speed blender.
Quickly combine until smooth.
Pour into a chilled glass and serve.
**Nutrition**:
Calories: 340  Fats: 11 g
Carbs: 48 g  Protein: 16 g

## 389. Roasted Asparagus

**Preparation Time: 10 minutes**
**Cooking Time: 10 minutes**
**Servings: 3**
**Ingredients:**

1 asparagus bunch, trimmed
3 tsp. avocado oil
A splash of lemon juice
Salt and ground black pepper to taste
1 tbsp. fresh oregano, chopped

**Directions:**
Spread the asparagus spears on a lined baking sheet, season with salt, and pepper, drizzle with oil and lemon juice, sprinkle with oregano, and toss to coat well.
Put in an oven at 425°F, and bake for 10 minutes.
Divide onto plates and serve.

**Nutrition**
Calories 130
Fat 1 g
Carbs 2 g
Protein 3 g

## 390. Asparagus Frittata
**Preparation Time: 10 minutes**
**Cooking Time: 15 minutes**
**Servings: 4**
**Ingredients:**
1/4 cup onion, chopped
Drizzle of olive oil
1-pound asparagus spears, cut into 1-inch pieces
Salt and ground black pepper to taste
4 eggs, whisked
1 cup cheddar cheese, grated

**Directions:**
Heat a pan with the oil over medium-high heat, add the onions, stir, and cook for 3 minutes. Add the asparagus, stir, and cook for 6 minutes. Add the eggs, stir, and cook for 3 minutes.
Add the salt and pepper sprinkle with the cheese, put in an oven, and broil for 3 minutes.
Divide the frittata onto plates and serve.

**Nutrition**
Calories 200

Fat 12 g
Carbs 5 g
Protein 14 g

## 391. Roasted Radishes
**Preparation Time: 10 minutes**
**Cooking Time: 35 minutes**
**Servings: 2**
**Ingredients:**
2 cups radishes cut in quarters
Salt and ground black pepper to taste
2 tbsp. butter, melted
1 tbsp. fresh chives, chopped
1 tbsp. lemon zest

**Directions:**
Spread the radishes on a lined baking sheet. Add the salt, pepper, chives, lemon zest, and butter, toss to coat, and bake in the oven at 375°F for 35 minutes.
Divide onto plates and serve.

**Nutrition:**
Calories 122
Fat 12 g
Carbs 3 g
Protein 14 g

## 392. Radish Hash Browns
**Preparation Time: 10 minutes.**
**Cooking Time: 10 minutes**
**Servings: 4**
**Ingredients:**
1/2 tsp. onion powder
1-pound radishes, shredded
1/2 tsp. garlic powder
Salt and ground black pepper to taste
4 eggs
1/3 Cup Parmesan cheese, grated

**Directions:**
In a bowl, mix the radishes with salt, pepper, onion, and garlic powder, eggs, and Parmesan cheese, and stir well.
Spread on a lined baking sheet, put in an oven at 375°F, and bake for 10

minutes. Divide the hash browns onto plates and serve.

**Nutrition:**
Calories 80  Fat 5 g
Carbs 5 g  Protein 7 g

## 393. Strawberry Frozen Yogurt

**Preparation Time: 10 minutes**
**Cooking Time: 15 minutes**
**Servings: 4**
**Ingredients:**
15 ounces of plain yogurt
6 ounces of strawberries
Juice of 1 orange
1 tablespoon honey
**Directions:**
Place the strawberries and orange juice into a food processor or blender and blitz until smooth.
Press the mixture through a sieve into a large bowl to remove seeds.
Stir in the honey and yogurt. Transfer the mixture to an ice-cream maker and follow the manufacturer's instructions.
Alternatively, pour the mixture into a container and place in the fridge for 1 hour. Use a fork to whisk it and break up the ice crystals and freeze for 2 hours.
**Nutrition:**
Calories: 238
Sodium: 33 mg
Dietary Fiber: 1.4 g
Total Fat: 1.8 g
Total Carbs: 12.3 g
Protein: 1.3 g

## 394. Walnut & Spiced Apple Tonic

**Preparation Time: 10 minutes**
**Cooking Time: 15 minutes**
**Servings: 1**
**Ingredients:**
6 walnuts halves

1 apple, cored
1 banana
1/2 teaspoon matcha powder
1/2 teaspoon cinnamon
Pinch of ground nutmeg

**Directions:**
Place ingredients into a blender and add sufficient water to cover them. Blitz until smooth and creamy.
**Nutrition:**
Calories: 124
Sodium: 22 mg
Dietary Fiber: 1.4 g
Total Fat: 2.1 g
Total Carbs: 12.3 g
Protein: 1.2 g

## 395. Basil & Walnut Pesto

**Preparation Time: 10 minutes**
**Cooking Time: 30 minutes**
**Servings: 1**
**Ingredients:**
2oz fresh basil
2oz walnuts
1oz pine nuts
3 cloves of garlic, crushed
2 tablespoons Parmesan, grated
4 tablespoons olive oil
**Direction**
Place the pesto ingredients into a food processor and process until it becomes a smooth paste.
Serve with meat, fish, salad and pasta dishes.
**Nutrition**
Calories: 136 Sodium: 23 mg,
Dietary Fiber: 1.2 g,
Total Fat: 3.1 g,  Total Carbs: 14.3 g
Protein: 1.4 g

## 396. Honey Chili Nuts

**Preparation Time: 10 minutes**
**Cooking Time: 30 minutes**
**Servings: 1**

**Ingredients:**
5oz walnuts
5oz pecan nuts
2oz softened butter
1 tablespoon honey
1/2 bird's-eye chili, very finely chopped and de-seeded
**Directions**
Preheat the oven to 180C/360F.
Combine the butter, honey and chili in a bowl, then add the nuts and stir them well.
Spread the nuts onto a lined baking sheet and roast them in the oven for 10 minutes, stirring once halfway through.
Remove from the oven and allow them to cool before eating.
**Nutrition:**
Calories: 295 Sodium: 28 mg
Dietary Fiber: 1.6 g
Total Fat: 4.7 g
Total Carbs: 14.6 g Protein: 1.3 g

## 397. Mozzarella Cauliflower Bars

**Preparation Time: 10 minutes**
**Cooking Time: 40 minutes**
**Servings: 12**
**Ingredients:**
1 big cauliflower head, riced
1/2 cup low-fat mozzarella cheese, shredded
1/4 cup egg whites
1 teaspoon Italian seasoning
Black pepper to the taste
**Directions:**
Spread the cauliflower rice on a lined baking sheet, cook in the oven at 375 degrees F for 20 minutes, transfer to a bowl, add black pepper, cheese, seasoning, and egg whites, stir well, spread into a rectangle pan and press on the bottom.

Introduce in the oven at 375 degrees F, bake for 20 minutes, cut into 12 bars, and serve as a snack.
**Nutrition:**
Calories 140 Fat 1 g
Carbohydrate 6 g
Protein 6 g

## 398. Grape, Celery & Parsley Reviver

**Preparation Time: 10 minutes**
**Cooking Time: 0 minutes**
**Servings: 2**
**Ingredients:**
75g 3ozred grapes
3 sticks of celery
1 avocado, de-stoned and peeled
1 tablespoon fresh parsley
1/2 teaspoon matcha powder
**Directions:**
Place all of the ingredients into a blender with enough water to cover them and blitz until smooth and creamy. Add crushed ice to make it even more refreshing.
**Nutrition:**
Calories 334
Fat 1.5 g
Carbohydrate 42.9 g
Protein 6 g

## 399. Roasted Red Endive With Caper Butter

**Preparation Time: 10 minutes**
**Cooking Time: 25 minutes**
**Servings: 4**
**Ingredients:**
10 – 12 red endives
2 teaspoons extra virgin olive oil
2–5 anchovy fillets, packed in oil
1 small lemon, juiced
3 tablespoons capers, drained
5 tablespoons cold butter, cut into cubes
1 tablespoon fresh parsley, chopped

Salt and pepper as needed
**Directions:**
Preheat the oven to 425 degrees F.
Toss endives with olive oil, salt, and pepper, and spread out on to a baking sheet cut side down. Bake for about 20-25 minutes or until caramelized.
While they're roasting, add the anchovies to a large pan over medium heat and use a fork to mash them until broken up.
Add lemon juice and mix well, then add capers.
Lower the heat and slowly stir in the butter and parsley.
Drizzle butter over roasted endives, season as necessary and garnish with more fresh parsley.
**Nutrition:**
Calories 109
Fat 8.6g
Protein1.5 g,
Carbohydrates 4.9 g,
Fiber 4 g

## 400. Zucchini Pepper Chips
**Preparation Time: 10 minutes**
**Cooking Time: 15 minutes**
**Servings: 04**
**Ingredients:**
1 2/3 cups vegetable oil
1 teaspoon garlic powder
1 teaspoon onion powder
1/2 teaspoon black pepper
3 tablespoons crushed red pepper flakes
2 zucchinis, thinly sliced
**Directions:**
Mix oil with all the spices in a bowl.
Add zucchini slices and mix well.
Transfer the mixture to a Ziplock bag and seal it.
Refrigerate for 10 minutes.
Spread the zucchini slices on a greased baking sheet.

Bake for 15 minutes
Serve.
**Nutrition:**
Calories 172  Total Fat 11.1 g
Saturated Fat 5.8 g
Cholesterol 610 mg   Sodium 749 mg
Total Carbs 19.9 g   Fiber 0.2 g
Sugar 0.2 g   Protein 13.5 g

## 401. Apple Chips
**Preparation Time: 15 Minutes**
**Cooking Time: 45 minutes**
**Servings:4**
**Ingredients:**
2 Golden Delicious apples, cored and thinly sliced
1 1/2 teaspoons white sugar
1/2 teaspoon ground cinnamon
**Directions:**
Set your oven to 225 degrees F.
Place apple slices on a baking sheet.
Sprinkle sugar an
d cinnamon over apple slices.
Bake for 45 minutes.
Serve
**Nutrition:**
Calories 127
Total Fat 3.5 g
Saturated Fat 0.5 g
Cholesterol 162 mg
Sodium 142 mg
Total Carbs 33.6g
Fiber 0.4 g
Sugar 0.5 g
Protein 4.5 g

## 402. Carrot Chips
**Preparation Time: 15 Minutes**
**Cooking Time: 12 minutes**
**Servings: 4**
**Ingredients:**
4 carrots, washed, peeled and sliced
2 teaspoons extra-virgin olive oil
1/4 teaspoon sea salt
**Directions:**

Set your oven to 350 degrees F.
Toss carrots with salt and olive oil.
Spread the slices on two baking sheets
in a single layer.
Bake for 6 minutes on upper and lower
rack of the oven.
Switch the baking racks and bake for
another 6 minutes.

Serve.
**Nutrition:**
Calories 153
Total Fat 7.5 g
Saturated Fat 1.1 g
Cholesterol 20 mg
Sodium 97 mg
Total Carbs 20.4 g
Fiber 0 g
Sugar 0 g
Protein 3.1g

## 403. Cinnamon Maple Sweet Potato Bites

**Preparation Time: 15 Minutes**
**Cooking Time: 25 minutes**
**Servings: 3–4**
**Ingredients:**
1/2 tsp. corn-starch
1 tsp. cinnamon
4 medium sweet potatoes, then peeled and cut into bite-size cubes
2–3 tbsp. maple syrup
3 tbsp. butter, melted
**Directions:**
Transfer the potato cubes to a bag Ziploc® and add in 3 tbsp. of melted butter. Seal and shake well until the potato cubes are coated with butter.
Add in the remaining ingredients and shake again.
Transfer the potato cubes to a parchment-lined baking sheet. The cubes shouldn't be stacked on one another.
Sprinkle with the cinnamon, if needed, and bake in a preheated oven at 425°F for about 25–30 minutes, stirring once during cooking.
Once done, take them out and stand them at room temperature. Enjoy!
**Nutrition:**
Calories: 436  Fats: 17.4 g
Carbs: 71.8 g
Protein: 4.1 g

## 404. Cheesy Kale Chips

**Preparation Time: 3 minutes**
**Cooking Time: 12 minutes**
**Servings: 4**
**Ingredients:**
3 tbsp. nutritional yeast
1 head curly kale, washed, ribs
3/4 tsp. garlic powder
1 tbsp. olive oil
1 tsp. onion powder
Salt, to taste
**Directions:**
Line cookie sheets with parchment paper.
Drain the kale leaves and tear them into chips, and spread them on the parchment paper.
Then, kindly transfer the leaves to a bowl and sized pieces
Add in 1 tsp. of onion powder, 3 tbsp. of nutritional yeast, 1 tbsp. of olive oil, and 3/4 tsp. of garlic powder. Mix with your hands.
Spread the kale onto prepared cookie sheets. They shouldn't touch each other.
Bake in a preheated oven at 350°F for about 10–12 minutes.
Once crisp, take out from the oven, and sprinkle with a bit of salt. Serve and enjoy!
**Nutrition:**
Calories: 71
Fats: 4 g
Carbs: 5 g
Protein: 4 g

## 405. Lemon Roasted Bell Pepper

**Preparation Time: 10 minutes**
**Cooking Time: 5 minutes**
**Servings: 4**
**Ingredients:**
4 bell peppers
1 tsp. olive oil

1 tbsp. mango juice

1/4 tsp. garlic, minced

1 tsp. oregano

1 pinch salt

1 pinch pepper

**Directions:**

Start heating the Air Fryer to 390°F.

Place some bell pepper in the air fryer.

Drizzle it with olive oil and air fry for 5 minutes.

Transfer it to a serving plate.

Take a small bowl and add the garlic, oregano, mango juice, salt, and pepper.

Mix them well and drizzle the mixture over the peppers.

Serve and enjoy!

**Nutrition:**

Calories: 59

Carbs: 6 g

Fats: 5 g

Protein: 4 g

## 406. Subtle Roasted Mushrooms

**Preparation Time: 10 minutes**

**Cooking Time: 5 minutes**

**Servings: 4**

**Ingredients:**

2 tsp. mixed Sebi-friendly herbs

1 tbsp. olive oil

1/2 tsp. garlic powder

2 lb. mushrooms

2 tbsp. date sugar

**Directions:**

Wash the mushrooms and turn dry in a plate of mixed greens spinner.

Quarter them and put them in a safe spot.

Put the garlic, oil, and spices in the dish of your oar-type air fryer.

Warmth for 2 minutes.

Stir it.

Add some mushrooms and cook for 25 minutes.

Then include vermouth and cook for 5 minutes more.

Serve and enjoy!

**Nutrition:**

Calories: 94

Carbs: 3 g

Fats: 8 g

Protein: 2 g

## 407. Kale Chips

**Preparation Time: 10 minutes**

**Cooking Time: 0 minutes**

**Servings: 1**

**Ingredients**

1 large bunch kale, washed and thoroughly dried, stems removed, leaves cut into 2-inch pieces

2 tablespoons extra-virgin olive oil

1 teaspoon sea salt

**Directions**

Preheat the oven to 275°F.

In a large bowl, use your hands to mix the kale and olive oil until the kale is evenly coated.

Transfer the kale to a large baking sheet and sprinkle the sea salt over it.

Bake, turning the kale leaves once halfway through, until crispy, about 20 minutes.

**Nutrition:**

Calories: 88

Total Fat: 7.2g

Total Carbohydrates: 5.7g

Sugar: 1.3g; Fiber: 2g

Protein: 1.9g

Sodium: 605mg

## 408. Chickpea Paste

**Preparation Time: 15 minutes**

**Cooking Time: 30 minutes**

**Servings: 1**

**Ingredients**

1 (15-ounce) can chickpeas, drained and rinsed

1/4 cup extra-virgin olive oil

1/4 cup fresh lemon juice
1/4 cup minced onion
1 garlic clove, minced
1 teaspoon sea salt
1/2 teaspoon ground cumin
1/4 teaspoon red pepper flakes

**Directions**

In a medium bowl, use a potato masher to mash the chickpeas until they are mostly broken up.

Add the olive oil, lemon juice, onion, garlic, salt, cumin, and red pepper flakes and continue mashing until you have a slightly chunky paste. Let sit for 30 minutes at room temperature for the flavors to develop, then serve.

**Nutrition:**
Calories: 110
Total Fat: 8g;
Total Carbohydrates: 10g
Sugar: 2g
Fiber: 2g
Protein: 3g
Sodium: 290mg

## 409. Spiced Nuts

**Preparation Time: 15 minutes**
**Cooking Time: 15 minutes**
**Servings:**
**Ingredients**
1 cup almonds
1/2 cup walnuts
1/4 cup sunflower seeds
1/4 cup pumpkin seeds
1 teaspoon ground turmeric
1/2 teaspoon ground cumin
1/4 teaspoon garlic powder
1/4 teaspoon red pepper flakes

**Directions**

Preheat the oven to 350°F.

Combine all the ingredients in a medium bowl and mix well.

Spread the nuts evenly on a rimmed baking sheet and bake until lightly toasted, 10 to 15 minutes.

Cool completely before serving or storing.

**Nutrition:**
Calories: 180
Total Fat: 16g
Total Carbohydrates: 7g
Sugar: 1g
Fiber: 3g
Protein: 6g
Sodium: 5g

## 410. Coconut-Mango Lassi

**Preparation Time: 10 minutes**
**Cooking Time: 0 minutes**
**Servings: 1**
**Ingredients**
11/2 cups frozen mango chunks
1 cup unsweetened coconut milk
1 cup ice cubes
1/2 cup plain yogurt
1 tablespoon honey
Pinch ground cardamom

**Directions**

Combine the mango, coconut milk, ice cubes, yogurt, and honey in a blender and blend until smooth.

Pour into two tall glasses. Sprinkle a little ground cardamom over each drink and serve.

**Nutrition:**
Calories: 370
Total Fat: 26g
Total Carbohydrates: 32g
Sugar: 27g
Fiber: 2g
Protein: 8g
Sodium: 30mg

## 411. Avocado Fudge

**Preparation Time: 10 minutes**
**Cooking Time: 0 minutes**
**Servings: 1**
**Ingredients**
11/2 cup bittersweet chocolate chips
1/4 cup coconut oil

1 ripe avocado, peeled and pitted
1/2 teaspoon sea salt

**Directions**

Line an 8-inch square baking pan with waxed or parchment paper.

In a double boiler (not the microwave), melt the chocolate and coconut oil.

Once melted, transfer to the bowl of a food processor and let them cool a bit. (If the chocolate is too hot when combined with the avocado, the mixture will separate.) Add the avocado and process until smooth.

Spoon the mixture into the lined pan, sprinkle with the sea salt, and chill for 3 hours. Cut into 16 pieces and serve.

**Nutrition:**
Calories: 120
Total Fat: 9g
Total Carbohydrates: 11g
Sugar: 9g
Fiber: 2g
Protein: 1g
Sodium: 80mg

## 412. Caramelized Pears With Yogurt

**Preparation Time: 10 minutes**
**Cooking Time: 5 minutes**
**Servings: 1**

**Ingredients**

1 tablespoon coconut oil
4 pears, peeled, cored, and quartered
2 tablespoons honey
1 teaspoon ground cinnamon
1/8 teaspoon sea salt
2 cups plain yogurt
1/4 cup chopped toasted pecans (optional)

**Directions**

Heat the oil in a large skillet over medium-high heat

Add the pears, honey, cinnamon, and salt, cover, and cook, stirring occasionally, until the fruit is tender, 4 to 5 minutes.

Uncover and let the sauce simmer for several more minutes to thicken.

Spoon the yogurt into four dessert bowls. Top with the warm pears, garnish with the pecans (if using), and serve.

**Nutrition:**

## 413. Almond Crackers

**Preparation Time: 15 minutes**
**Cooking Time: 20 minutes**
**Servings: 2**

Ingredients

1 cup almond flour
1/4 teaspoon baking soda
1/4 teaspoon salt
1/8 teaspoon black pepper
3 tablespoons sesame seeds
1 egg, beaten
Salt and pepper to taste

**Directions**

Preheat your oven to 350 °F

Line two baking sheets with parchment paper and keep them on the side

Mix the dry ingredients into a large bowl and add egg, mix well and form a dough

Divide dough into two balls

Roll out the dough between two pieces of parchment paper

Cut into crackers and transfer them to prep a baking sheet

Bake for 15-20 minutes

Repeat until all the dough has been used up

Leave crackers to cool and serve

**Nutrition:**
Calories: 302
Fat: 28g
Carbohydrates: 4g

Protein: 9g

# CHAPTER 16:

# Desserts

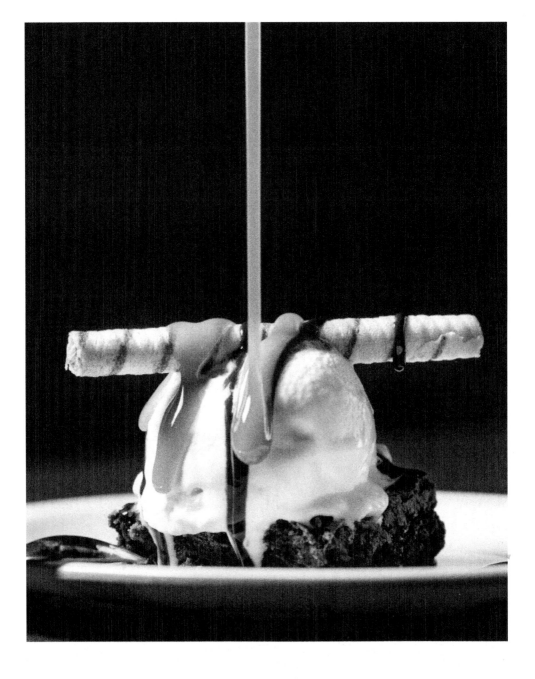

## 414. Cardamom Tart
**Preparation Time: 10 minutes**
**Cooking Time: 10 minutes**
**Servings: 8**
**Ingredients**
4-5 pears
2 tablespoons lemon juice
pastry sheets
**CARDAMOMO FILLING**
1/2 lb. butter
1/2 lb. brown sugar
1/2 lb. almonds
1/4 lb. flour
1 1/4 tsp cardamom
2 eggs
**Directions**
Preheat oven to 400 F, unfold pastry sheets and place them on a baking sheet
Toss together all ingredients together and mix well
Spread mixture in a single layer on the pastry sheets
Before baking decorate with your desired fruits and bake for 10 minutes
**Nutrition:**
calories 270
fat 10
fiber 3
carbs 12
protein 31

## 415. Pear Tart
**Preparation Time: 10 minutes**
**Cooking Time: 25 minutes**
**Servings: 1**
**Ingredients**
1 lb. pears
2 oz. brown sugar
1/2 lb. flaked almonds
1/4 lb. porridge oat
2 oz. flour
1/4 lb. almonds
pastry sheets

2 tablespoons syrup

**Directions**
Preheat oven to 400 F, unfold pastry sheets and place them on a baking sheet
Toss together all ingredients together and mix well
Spread mixture in a single layer on the pastry sheets
Before baking decorate with your desired fruits
Bake at 400 F for 22-25 minutes or until golden brown
When ready remove from the oven and serve
**Nutrition:**
Calories: 310
Protein: 49.7g
Fat: 6.8g
Carbs: 8.4g

## 416. Peach Pecan Pie
**Preparation Time: 10 minutes**
**Cooking Time: 30 minutes**
**Servings: 4**
**Ingredients**
4-5 cups peaches
1 tablespoon preserves
1 cup sugar
4 small egg yolks
1/4 cup flour
1 tsp vanilla extract
**Directions**
Line a pie plate or pie form with pastry and cover the edges of the plate depending on your preference
In a bowl combine all pie ingredients together and mix well
Pour the mixture over the pastry
Bake at 400-425 F for 25-30 minutes or until golden brown
When ready remove from the oven and let it rest for 15 minutes
**Nutrition:**

calories 71 fat 1.6
fiber 2.1 carbs 12.8 protein 2.3

## 417. Butterfinger Pie

**Preparation Time: 10 minutes**
**Cooking Time: 30 minutes**
**Servings: 9**
**Ingredients**
pastry sheets
1 package cream cheese
1 tsp vanilla extract
1/4 cup peanut butter
1 cup powdered sugar (to decorate)
2 cups Butterfinger candy bars
8 oz whipped topping
**Directions**
Line a pie plate or pie form with pastry and cover the edges of the plate depending on your preference
In a bowl combine all pie ingredients together and mix well
Pour the mixture over the pastry
Bake at 400-425 F for 25-30 minutes or until golden brown
When ready remove from the oven and let it rest for 15 minutes
**Nutrition:**
242 Calories  25g carbs
12g fat
13g protein

## 418. Strawberry Pie

**Preparation Time: 10 minutes**
**Cooking Time: 30 minutes**
**Servings: 8**
**Ingredients**
 pastry sheets
1,5 lb. strawberries
1 cup powdered sugar
2 tablespoons cornstarch
1 tablespoon lime juice
1 tsp vanilla extract - 2 eggs
2 tablespoons butter
**Directions**

Line a pie plate or pie form with pastry and cover the edges of the plate depending on your preference
In a bowl combine all pie ingredients together and mix well
Pour the mixture over the pastry
Bake at 400-425 F for 25-30 minutes or until golden brown
When ready remove from the oven and let it rest for 15 minutes
**Nutrition:**
calories 200 fat 6 fiber 3.4
carbs 7.6 protein 3

## 419. Pistachios Ice Cream

**Preparation Time: 10 minutes**
**Cooking Time: 0 minutes**
**Servings: 7**
**Ingredients**
4 egg yolks
 1 cup heavy cream
 1 cup milk
1 cup sugar
1 vanilla bean
1 tsp almond extract
1 cup cherries
1/2 cup pistachios
**Directions**
In a saucepan whisk together all ingredients
Mix until bubbly
Strain into a bowl and cool
Whisk in favorite fruits and mix well
Cover and refrigerate for 2-3 hours
Pour mixture in the ice-cream maker and follow manufacturer instructions
Serve when ready
**Nutrition:**
Calories: 371 Carbs: 15.5 g
Protein: 62 g;

## 420. Vanilla Ice Cream

**Preparation Time: 10 minutes**
**Cooking Time: 0 minutes**
**Servings: 1**

## Ingredients

1 cup milk
1 tablespoon cornstarch
1 oz. cream cheese
1 cup heavy cream
1 cup brown sugar
1 tablespoon corn syrup
1 vanilla bean

## Directions

In a saucepan whisk together all ingredients
Mix until bubbly
Strain into a bowl and cool
Whisk in favorite fruits and mix well
Cover and refrigerate for 2-3 hours
Pour mixture in the ice-cream maker and follow manufacturer instructions
Serve when ready

## Nutrition:

448 Calories
27g fat
41g carbs
15g protein

## 421. Cashew Almond Butter

**Preparation Time: 10 minutes**
**Cooking Time: 12 minutes**
**Servings: 1**

## Ingredients

1 cup almonds, blanched
1/3 cup cashew nuts
2 tablespoons coconut oil
Salt as needed
1/2 teaspoon cinnamon

## Directions

Preheat your oven to 350 °F
Bake almonds and cashews for 12 minutes
Let them cool
Transfer to a food processor and add remaining ingredients
Add oil and keep blending until smooth
Serve and enjoy!

## Nutrition:

Fat: 19g
Carbohydrates: 205g
Protein: 2.8g

## 422. Nut and Chia Mix

**Preparation Time: 10 minutes**
**Cooking Time: 0 minutes**
**Servings: 1**

## Ingredients

1-ounce hazelnuts
1 tablespoon chia seeds
2 cups of water
1-ounce Macadamia nuts
1-2 packets Stevia, optional

## Directions

Add all the listed ingredients to a blender. Blend on high until smooth and creamy. Enjoy your smoothie.

## Nutrition:

Fat: 43g
Carbohydrates: 15g
Protein: 9g

## 423. Easy Fudge

**Preparation Time: 10 minutes**
**Cooking Time: 0 minutes**
**Servings: 2**

## Ingredients

1 3/4 cups of coconut butter
1 cup pumpkin puree
1 teaspoon ground cinnamon
1/4 teaspoon ground nutmeg
1 tablespoon coconut oil

## Directions

Take an 8x8 inch square baking pan and line it with aluminum foil
Take a spoon and scoop out the coconut butter into a heated pan and allow the butter to melt
Keep stirring well and remove from the heat once fully melted
Add spices and pumpkin and keep straining until you have a grain-like texture

Add coconut oil and keep stirring to incorporate everything

Scoop the mixture into your baking pan and evenly distribute it

Place wax paper on top of the mixture and press gently to straighten the top

Remove the paper and discard

Allow it to chill for 1-2 hours

Once chilled, take it out and slice it up into pieces

**Nutrition:**
Calories: 120
Fat: 10g Carbohydrates: 5g
Protein: 1.2g

## 424. The Coconut Loaf
**Preparation Time: 10 minutes**
**Cooking Time: 0 minutes**
**Servings: 2**
**Ingredients**
1 1/2 tablespoons coconut flour
1/4 teaspoon baking powder
1/8 teaspoon salt
1 tablespoon coconut oil, melted
1 whole egg
**Directions**
Preheat your oven to 350 °F

Add coconut flour, baking powder, salt

Add coconut oil, eggs and stir well until mixed

Leave the batter for several minutes

Pour half the batter onto the baking pan

Spread it to form a circle, repeat with remaining batter

Bake in the oven for 10 minutes

Once a golden-brown texture comes, let it cool and serve

**Nutrition:**
Calories: 297
Fat: 14g
Carbohydrates: 15g
Protein: 15g

## 425. Chocolate Parfait
**Preparation Time: 10 minutes**
**Cooking Time: 0 minutes**
**Servings: 1**
**Ingredients**
2 tablespoons cocoa powder
1 cup almond milk
1 tablespoon chia seeds
Pinch of salt
1/2 teaspoon vanilla extract
**Directions**
Take a bowl and add cocoa powder, almond milk, chia seeds, vanilla extract, and stir

Transfer to dessert glass and place in your fridge for 2 hours

**Nutrition:**
Calories: 130
Fat: 5g
Carbohydrates: 7g
Protein: 16g

# Measurement Conversion Tables

## Volume Equivalents (Liquid)

| US STANDARD | US STANDARD (OUNCES) | METRIC (APPROXIMATE) |
|---|---|---|
| 2 tablespoons | 1 fl. oz. | 30 mL |
| 1/4 cup | 2 fl. oz. | 60 mL |
| 1/2 cup | 4 fl. oz. | 120 mL |
| 1 cup | 8 fl. oz. | 240 mL |
| 1-1/2 cups | 12 fl. oz. | 355 mL |
| 2 cups or 1 pint | 16 fl. oz. | 475 mL |
| 4 cups or 1 quart | 32 fl. oz. | 1 L |
| 1 gallon | 128 fl. oz. | 4 L |

## Volume Equivalents (Dry)

| US STANDARD | METRIC (APPROXIMATE) |
|---|---|
| 1/8 teaspoon | 0.5 mL |
| 1/4 teaspoon | 1 mL |
| 1/2 teaspoon | 2 mL |
| 3/4 teaspoon | 4 mL |
| 1 teaspoon | 5 mL |
| 1 tablespoon | 15 mL |
| 1/4 cup | 59 mL |
| 1/3 cup | 79 mL |
| 1/2 cup | 118 mL |
| 2/3 cup | 156 mL |
| 3/4 cup | 177 mL |
| 1 cup | 235 mL |
| 2 cups or 1 pint | 475 mL |
| 3 cups | 700 mL |
| 4 cups or 1 quart | 1 L |

## Oven Temperatures

| FAHRENHEIT (F) | CELSIUS (C) (APPROXIMATE) |
| --- | --- |
| 250° | 120° |
| 300° | 150° |
| 325° | 165° |
| 350° | 180° |
| 375° | 190° |
| 400° | 200° |
| 425° | 220° |
| 450° | 230° |

## Weight Equivalents

| US STANDARD | METRIC (APPROXIMATE) |
| --- | --- |
| 1/2 ounce | 15 g |
| 1 ounce | 30 g |
| 2 ounces | 60 g |
| 4 ounces | 115 g |
| 8 ounces | 225 g |
| 12 ounces | 340 g |
| 16 ounces or 1 pound | 455 g |

# Conclusion

Thank you reading this book. This book is meant for those that have a relative or friend suffering from a fatty liver and want to understand this condition. I assume you already have such an overview, if you are suffering from it yourself. This book has explained everything you can do to take away accumulated fat in your liver as well as remove harmful deposits in it such as gallbladder stones. These are information you should know of so that you would be able to determine if you are suffering from this condition. If you know what you are experiencing, you can prevent the disease from worsening and ultimately this book provides proven steps to cure fatty liver for life.

Excessive calories can make fat build up in your liver and the latter will then have a hard time to perform its function which is to break fats down. Overconsumption of alcohol can also make fat accumulate in your liver. Genetics is also a possible cause.

If you fail to treat liver diseases such as a fatty liver, this organ will become scarred and hardened and you will suffer from a serious condition called cirrhosis. Eventually, cirrhosis will result to liver failure. This condition has a few symptoms so you may not see signs of having it.

The Liver Cleanse is a way of decongesting your liver, the bile ducts that are critical to its functions and your colon immediately. With a process that only lasts from the evening of one day to the morning of the next, you can get rid of the gallstones obstructing your system. And yes, you still get your regular eight-hour sleep.

Ingredients introduced to the system during the flush will soften and breakdown the gallstones. They'll dilate and oil the bile ducts to ensure the now softened gallstones travel through the body with as little drama as possible. It is an easy, pain-free, and safe process that will leave you feeling like a new person.

The effects of the Liver Cleanse are almost immediate. You will feel the immediate rejuvenation of your system. Your digestive system will be cleaned out. Your blood will be purified. The hormones in your body will be balanced better and your cells will be able to regenerate faster. You will look, feel and be better!

Everyone should do a Liver Cleanse at least once in their lifetime if not more. The benefits that come with it are incredible. Think of your body as a car that requires frequent servicing to increase its capacity to perform. Like servicing, the Liver Cleanse will energize and revitalize you, and ultimately increase your life expectancy. If you follow the instructions for both the preparation week and the overnight flush, precisely as prescribed, you'll be well on your way to better health.

Of course, not everyone will be open-minded to the process but none of the ingredients used are in any way harmful and the results afterwards speak for themselves.

Good luck.

# Index

Printed in Great Britain
by Amazon

78139092R00149